PRAISE FOR DEATH OF A THOUSAND CUTS

"I am so grateful for what this book could mean to women. It's sad to think about the hundreds of thousands of women who need this. My wish is that it gets into all of their hands. Thank you for writing it 🙏." —Alisa

"I think this book is going to connect with many on a deep level. Thank you for putting to words what I so closely experienced and identify with. There is something so powerful that happens when those who had a similar experience can relate. It un-silences something no one wants to hear about and makes you feel like you matter. It is life-saving work. Thank you Patrick for all you do." —Amy

"I loved it!!! I kept making stars* and highlights for myself and my kids. this will help so many people!" —Loretta

"Patrick's book takes the reader through elements of self-discovery via chapters on clarity, acceptance, truth, grief, detoxification, boundaries and new standards, to name a few. *Death of a Thousand Cuts* is an adult primer for the emotionally and spiritually abused that teaches you to know your intrinsic value and to let go of hope-ium and harm!" —Deb

"What I love about the book is that it's direct, clear, easy to understand, sound, and . . . well just downright awesome. The sections on breaking the rules of the system and the Committee in Your Mind are so spot on. So glad you've got a chapter on setting boundaries. Also, the section on relational parenting—so essential . . . so foundational . . . and shared just in the right place in the book. And the closing piece on presence and the Eugene Peterson visit was so beautiful." —Chris

"I love how the book sounds very much like Patrick in person, just like he's talking to you. It expresses his care and value of the reader, while at the same time speaks the truth very directly and clearly, which helps break the mental and emotional fog that so heavily contributes to the denial in women who have been abused. Makes our bruised souls finally feel heard." —Heather

Death of a Thousand Cuts:
The Impact of Emotional Abuse

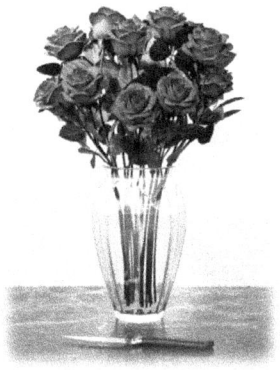

A Guide to Clarity and Healing
Patrick Doyle

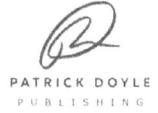

PATRICK DOYLE
PUBLISHING

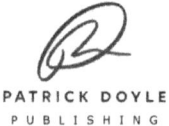

PATRICK DOYLE
PUBLISHING

Copyright © 2024 by Patrick Doyle
All rights reserved.
Published by Patrick Doyle Publishing
Jacksonville, OR

No portion of this book may be reproduced, stored in a retrieval system, or transmitted in any form or by any means—electronic, mechanical, photocopy, recording, scanning, or other—except for brief quotations in critical reviews or articles, without the prior written permission of the publisher. Although the publisher and the author have made every effort to ensure that the information in this book was correct at press time and while this publication is designed to provide accurate information in regard to the subject matter covered, the publisher and the author assume no responsibility for errors, inaccuracies, omissions, or any other inconsistencies herein and hereby disclaim any liability to any party for any loss, damage, or disruption caused by errors or omissions, whether such errors or omissions result from negligence, accident, or any other cause. This publication is meant as a source of valuable information for the reader, however it is not meant as a substitute for direct expert assistance. If such level of assistance is required, the services of a competent professional should be sought.

For information about special discounts for bulk purchases or author interviews, appearances, and speaking engagements please contact:

www.PatrickDoyle.life

First Edition

ISBN eBook	979-8-9911718-0-9
ISBN Paperback	979-8-9911718-1-6
ISBN Hardcover	979-8-9911718-2-3

Library of Congress: 2024917944

Edited by Jenna Love Schrader
Cover design by Patrick Feld
Book, page, jacket design, produced by Rodney Miles

It is in the whole process of meeting and solving problems that life has meaning. Problems are the cutting edge that distinguishes between success and failure. Problems call forth our courage and our wisdom; indeed, they create our courage and our wisdom. It is only because of problems that we grow mentally and spiritually. It is through the pain of confronting and resolving problems that we learn.

—M. Scott Peck[1]

*This book is dedicated
to all of the brave and courageous
survivors of abusive relationships.*

NOTE TO READERS

IN THIS BOOK I most often talk in terms of a marriage or an intimate relationship, or even more specifically of a *man* being abusive. The principles discussed here work nonetheless in other types of scenarios, but for the sake of clarity and as is most commonly discussed in the Pathway to Hope support group, I'm using them in this context. Other areas these principles can help resolve include parenting, child relationships, boss and employee relationships, other family situations, and so many more.

Please, whatever your situation, consider the world around you with the "new eyes" you might acquire as a result of reading this book. It's my experience through all my years of consulting that these principles have many and various uses, and all lead to freedom for you. And thanks, in advance, for reading.

—Patrick Doyle

CONTENTS

Note to Readers ix
Contents xi

Introduction: My Story of Abuse 1
    The Church's Divorce from Me 10
    My Divorce from the God I Thought I Knew 11

Section I: Become Clear 13
[1]   What is Emotional Abuse? 15
    What I Hear 18
    Some Reasons for the "Crazy" 19
    Document 21
    The Church and Emotional Abuse 22
[2]   What is Spiritual Abuse? 29
    Marriage as an Idol 34

[3] Codependency is External Dependance 41
How External Dependance Mixes with Emotional Abuse 42
The Origin of External Dependence 43
Benefits of *Not* Being Externally Dependent 44
[4] Clearing & Creating Internal Strength 47
Core Concepts for Transformational Power 48
Healthy Anger 56

Section II: Find Real Hope 61

[5] The Truth About Trust & Healing 63
Reconciliation or Rebuilding Trust 64
What is Your Gut Telling You? 65
When Your Abuser Has an Epiphany 67
Changed Behavior and the Church 69
Forgiveness and Healing 70
Putting It All Together 73
The First Step to Valuing Yourself 76
[6] What is Hope-ium? 77
Dealers 80
Acceptance 80
Living in the Truth 82
How to Live in the Truth 86

Giving CPR to a Dead Guy 87

Not Your Responsibility 91

[7] Grief & Documentation 95

Document Your Grief 99

The Committee in Your Mind 102

What Should I Document? 104

Why is Grief Important? 106

Riding the Waves of Grief 106

Things You Might Be Grieving 108

How Can I Tell if I am Avoiding Grief? 110

Who is the Person Responsible for Defining the Grief? 111

Will My Life Fall Apart if I Start to Grieve? 112

[8] Detox 115

Trust Your Gut 118

[9] How to Set Boundaries You Can Keep 123

What a Boundary Looks Like & How to Set One 124

Assess Your Safety Level 129

Section III: Live Free 135

[10] Intrinsic Value 137

You Are Valuable. 137

The Choices Are YOURS 142

[11] New Standards 143
    Relationships Post-Abuse 145
    Healthy Intimacy 147
[12] Relational Parenting 153
    Tell the Truth 155
    Magical Thinking 156
    Be Present 157
    Face Reality 158
    Drop It and Roll 159
    No Unsolicited Advice 160
    In Conclusion 163

Epilogue: The Power of Presence 165
About the Author 169
Glossary 173
Learn More 177
Notes 179

INTRODUCTION:

MY STORY OF ABUSE

MY ABUSE BEGAN in early childhood at the hands of my alcoholic parents. My dad was a veteran of two wars and a victim of post-traumatic stress disorder (PTSD). He was a dangerous, terrifying person to be around, especially as a child. Whenever something set him off, there would be a verbal tirade or a physical beating—often both.

My mom spent most of her time in her swivel chair in front of the TV. The dog would loyally sit next to her in the chair. The side table held an ashtray and her drink. Rock, smoke, drink, watch TV. That was her coping ritual. I have no memories of ever doing anything with my mom, not even grocery shopping.

DEATH OF A THOUSAND CUTS

Her life ended when I was ten years old. She died on Christmas Day as a result of her drinking. I was awash in pain and confusion. My young mind could not comprehend why God would take my mom away from me. In essence, I felt God had abandoned me to live with an irrational, crazy alcoholic father. It took me many years to forgive God for leaving me to be raised by a rabid wolf, so to speak.

I lived on high alert and learned to immediately gauge my dad's state of mind every time he entered a room.

Can I smell any alcohol on him?

Are his eyes bloodshot or clear?

Can he walk through the door without staggering?

I became adept at reading my dad's body language. I was in a constant state of trying to anticipate what he may or may not do. No child should have to live like that. Even a child as attentive as I had to be can never fully understand how dangerous it is to live with an alcoholic dealing with—or rather *not* dealing with—PTSD.

Around the age of twelve, my anger from the emotional and physical abuse I endured reached a fever pitch. I went to the library to research how I could *poison* my dad. I wanted the emotional and physical pain to stop. I was desperate, and him being gone seemed the best solution from my physical and emotional pain.

INTRODUCTION: MY STORY OF ABUSE

Before you report me to the FBI, rest assured that I never did anything of the sort, but I certainly thought long and hard about harming him. The survival instinct is real, and anyone experiencing that level of pain and abuse over a long period of time often has the very same thoughts. The flip side of feeling like I would do anything to survive was that I often felt deviant. Let me reassure you of something: Extreme survival fantasies and the impulse for self-preservation are normal reactions to abuse. How else should one respond to levels of injustice that are endlessly inflicted by a parental figure?

How does one cope, at the age of ten, with their mom's death and being left alone to live—or should I say *survive*?—with an extremely violent dad? Well, I smoked pot to cope. Did it help? It helped enough for me to keep doing it. By age twelve I was actually dreaming of leading my own drug cartel someday.

Drug use did not work in my favor, though, when I went to live with my sister at the age of thirteen. In fact, I was so difficult for her to manage, she sent me back to live with my dad after only two years. By the time I was sixteen, I was on my way to fulfilling my dream of leading a drug cartel and making enough money from selling drugs to live in my own apartment. However, skimming money off the top from the drugs I sold for a mob guy was *not* a good idea. One day, he showed up at my apartment, pointed a gun at my head, and threatened to take my life. Needless to say, that was the end of my drug career—thankfully!

DEATH OF A THOUSAND CUTS

Following that life-threatening event, I did not want to go back and live with my dad. On November 7, 1980, still only sixteen, I ended up on my sister and brother-in-law's doorstep again, only three years after I had been kicked out. I was not a healthy soul at the time, and I was grateful they decided to take me back.

The first weekend I was there, I went to church with my sister and her husband. What do you think happened? Lo and behold, I was "saved." The only thought running through my mind was, *I'm a Jesus person now!*

An indescribable kind of love that I had never felt or sensed before overpowered my being. It was the beginning of my soul transformation. I soon realized that being loved was what the people in the church were all talking about when I'd sit and listen to the sermons and hear the chatter in the lobby. To be loved was what I desired more than anything. I realized I was no different than anyone else. All humans are wired for giving and receiving love. It was simply withheld from me in my formative years. Specifically, I had to come into the understanding of *agape love*[2], which transcends and persists unconditionally and is the highest form of love we can experience. It took me a while to accept and feel worthy of such a gift.

I didn't doubt the love I was feeling. It was real, and I was seeing it play out in my small world. Despite my experiences, I still felt shame. I call it a "shame frame" that was instilled in me from a very early age. My shame frame told me that if I didn't perform exactly the way my dad required me to perform, I

INTRODUCTION: MY STORY OF ABUSE

would get in trouble, which meant a verbal and/or physical assault. My dad had been in the military and was used to receiving orders and being berated at times because that is the general climate. This military practice is done with the mindset of training mentally strong and disciplined soldiers, but raising children in this manner is cruel and emotionally harmful.

In my early childhood, inspections were an everyday occurrence. My room was a replica of an Army barrack. I had a military bunk made with a steel frame and steel springs; a thin, uncomfortable mattress; and a U.S. Army blanket that had to be perfectly centered on the bed, tucked in, and clean. My room could not have a trace of dust anywhere or else I got in big "trouble." Here is an example of how my early years looked: Perform as Dad says, and you won't get a beating. Screw up, and you will receive a beating, be it verbal and/or physical. The emotional fallout for *not performing* showed up as humiliation and shame.

Since my early experiences were viewed through my lens, it became the only lens I knew. As a result, I couldn't help but feel that God was looking at me through the same "shame frame" lens. Any child would be susceptible to this faulty set of beliefs: *You're not good enough. You are unworthy of love. You can't do anything right. You must be punished for being so stupid and incompetent.*

The original message I heard at church was, "God loves you. Come as you are. He is full of grace and mercy. He wants you to be in His family. He cares about you. He knows everything."

Don't misunderstand what I'm saying. All of those statements are true. But don't forget that I was hearing everything through my "shame frame" lens.

Six months *after* my salvation, I was asked, "Have you been praying? Are you serving? Are you tithing? Are you reading the Bible?" Suddenly, God's love no longer seemed merciful and free. In fact, it seemed like I was only loved if I performed according to a set of rules, which made me have flashbacks to life with my dad.

My fear-based response, when faced with Christianity or going back to my childhood home? *I can be a good soldier! I know how to do that! If I follow God, then He will love and bless me!*

So I performed and became a very good Christian. I fasted. I tithed. I went to church regularly. I read and memorized the Bible. I even began a career in ministry because I believed that was where my value came from. Eventually, that belief became true for me. My value was equal to how well I served in the church. I became deeply involved in my career and service within the church. As a result, my shame became spiritualized.

And then I got married.

Marriage is already complicated for "normal" people, let alone for those who have trauma embedded within them from years of abuse, which was my personal brand of trauma. Not only was I abused emotionally and physically, but I had never *seen* what a healthy marriage looked like. So when I got married, there was trouble right from the get-go. I immediately started to hear a language that is particular to manipulators,

INTRODUCTION: MY STORY OF ABUSE

though I was unfamiliar with the strategies used on me. I was so used to cruelty and being told what to do or how to correct my behavior that I was blinded for many years in my marriage.

"I'm sorry, but *you* never said that!"

"I wouldn't have done *that* if *you* hadn't done *this*."

Everything was my responsibility and my fault. As a result, I felt crazy and was always pegged as being the one with the problem. I was certain there was something wrong with me. *Why can't I do anything right?* was constantly streaming through my thoughts. No matter how many times I tried to resolve something, nothing would change. To my wife, I was the problem, and I alone held the solution. But again, no matter how I adjusted myself, there was never any solution. Thus began a never-ending cycle of shame and failure.

I'm not saying I was a perfect partner. And despite the fact that most of you reading this are probably women, in this case I'm talking about my (former) abusive wife. It was an eye-opening experience for me. I just want to be clear about this because I have found most women who are being abused are actually being accused of being abusive themselves, a lie which is part of the abuse! And there is a big difference between being wrongly accused of being abusive, and actually being abusive.

My religious beliefs and position as a pastor and Christian TV radio personality in the community created a lot of internal pressure to pretend that things weren't as bad as they were. I also believed that it was my job alone to keep everything together. There were many times I felt like I needed to leave the relationship, but the stigma of ending the marriage contract and leaving felt like a death sentence for my career, my friendships, and my future. Each time I would plan on leaving, I would always go back because I thought that was what God wanted me to do.

> *Each time I would plan on leaving,*
> *I would always go back*
> *because I thought that was what*
> *God wanted me to do.*

After twenty-five years of marriage, I finally initiated a separation. While in counseling during our separation, my therapist helped me to understand this faulty reasoning by explaining it to me this way: "The Spirit was urging you to leave the harmful relationship, yet your religious, shame-based fear was pushing you back into that harmful relationship." In other words, I was learning how to manage my abuse. My "normal" relationship style was to be abused, therefore walking away from the marriage felt uncomfortable and unnatural. In reality, though, my discomfort was the Spirit all along trying to move me.

What's ironic is that I was counseling many people during this confusing era of transformation that was paired with stops and starts. I was the director of treatment agencies that specifically worked with drug and alcohol programs, intervening in people's lives, and helping them become aware

INTRODUCTION: MY STORY OF ABUSE

of the reasoning behind their actions and destructive patterns. Daily, I was guiding people out of situations and conditions that resulted in emotional abuse and then offering life-changing treatments for that abuse. Unfortunately, in my own life, I was in deep denial, and that denial created the blinders that kept me managing the abuse rather than overcoming it.

When I finally realized I did have a problem, I had already planted a church, started a movie company, and was on the TV and radio. I was Patrick Doyle, the emotional abuse expert! I was the guy who helped people heal or remove themselves from toxic relationships! Well, the truth is, I *am* an emotional abuse expert because I've lived through the experience more than once and have come out the other side each time. I understand the denial people experience because I once denied my own relationship realities.

I finally knew that the toxic relationship I was in was not something God wanted for me. Divorce is difficult for anyone, but often it brings relief. My divorce relieved me of the toxic place I felt was my duty to remain in. Post-divorce life made me feel alive because it was the first time in my life I was free from abuse. However, my divorce brought with it losses I did not anticipate. I call these losses my secondary divorces. Why? Because I lost countless friends, my identity, my family, my church, and the God that I had come to know up until that point.

DEATH OF A THOUSAND CUTS

The Church's Divorce from Me

After years of counseling people who had been harmed in the church because of the institution's neglect and failure of handling painful and difficult circumstances, I realized what people needed were not platitudes, to-do lists, and Scripture verses. What they needed was a safe, relational connection. This inspired me to start a new kind of church based on what I had come to value most: authentic relationships.

Developing intimate relationships had always been my goal while working in the church. As a result, deep and meaningful connections were made, people felt safe to be themselves, and I witnessed more healing occurring than harm.

When I got divorced, I did not anticipate the people whom I had personally helped abandoning and judging me. The truth is, the people I considered my brothers, sisters, and friends believed the rumors and slander. Why? Because of the conflict of their belief structure that divorce is wrong, no matter the sobering facts surrounding the situation. They believed the slander because it was too difficult to accept the truth of what was actually happening. Despite the years of behavioral evidence in my relationships with each one of these people, they chose to believe the lies of the person (my ex-wife) who displayed years of harmful behavior, which many observed firsthand.

I wasn't abandoned by a group, per se, but by many individuals whom I had intimate relationships with for years. My divorce proved that I was, as my father had shown,

INTRODUCTION: MY STORY OF ABUSE

dismissible and disrespected. I became a *persona non grata*—an "unwelcome and or unacceptable person" in the worst sense of the term. I was merely "someone they used to know" in the best sense. I went from community hero to community zero. The pain of that rejection from the people in the church whom I thought cared about me led me to question my beliefs about God.

My Divorce from the God I Thought I Knew

The God I knew was built on thirty years of studying the Bible and theology, engaging in church leadership, and pastoring. I was deeply invested in the principles I believed God wanted me to live by. The directives I was given by the church and the way the Bible was translated and explained to me by my original teachers and mentors became the foundation of my life, not something ancillary to it. The God I knew formed the basis on how I chose to live in the world, survive in the world, and interact with the world. The church was the only safe place I had known. It was also the foundation of my career as a "biblical counselor." My beliefs formed the foundation of my entire existence. The pain of losing my close relationships and the rejection I lived through did not match the beliefs I had based my life on.

While in deep grief from the pain of losing my marriage, I found no comfort from the church, intimate friendships, family, or my beliefs for the first time in my life. I clearly remember one light emerging: In the midst of my soul-crushing grief, I was visited by the Spirit. This encounter kept me from being destroyed by the onslaught of suffering and rejection. I soon came to realize that the many things I spent years teaching people about weren't working for me anymore. It was like I was on a small boat in the middle of a vast ocean in the pitch-black night with no oar, no motor, and no sail. Nothing! I sat there all alone, not knowing where I was going or how to get there. This is what I recall being the first step in deconstructing my old belief systems. I felt lonely, troubled, uncertain, unprepared, abandoned, and clueless.

You may be at a point in your life where you need to be really honest with yourself and brave enough to gain a perspective and adopt a tireless hope that says, "It's time to move forward in your life." Getting out of an abusive relationship can be difficult for many reasons. Maybe your marriage isn't as bad as the childhood you endured. Or maybe your marriage isn't as bad as someone else's. But those excuses should not be your guiding factor. What *matters* is if your marriage is bad for *you*. Perhaps you feel you're just too weak, but maybe you can get out for your kids' sake. If that's your motivation, then good! I don't care what the motive is, as long as you find one. You are not going to heal from the abuse by avoiding it.

When you start to confront the abuse, it's going to get messy, but the mess is going to lead to healing, and that's the main goal for you now. I'm on the other side, and you can get there, too.

SECTION I:
BECOME CLEAR

DEATH OF A THOUSAND CUTS

[1]

WHAT IS EMOTIONAL ABUSE?

OVER THE YEARS, there have been many definitions of *emotional abuse*. Based on my years of experience, my definition of abuse is when one person in a relationship is being repeatedly harmed and destroyed by the other person—emotionally, physically, and/or spiritually. Abuse happens when the abuser participates in behaviors that leave the victim feeling responsible for all the problems while simultaneously never allowing for resolution, no matter what the abused person tries or suggests. This is because the abuser has such intact and high levels of denial. Their denial is so deep that they believe their own lies. Thus, an abuser can lie to a person's face

DEATH OF A THOUSAND CUTS

and be shocked and hurt when that person doesn't believe them.

This is also why they are generally well-liked by others, which causes more confusion for the victim. Therefore an abuser can make anything true, no matter the facts. This denial is the reason they make their partners sick—in mind and body. Denial is also the reason that nothing gets resolved. The one being harmed is blamed and then made to believe there is something wrong with them. The cycle of abuse becomes normalized after time, leaving the abused to question their own reality.

The abuser uses the following tactics:

- Rationalizing
- Minimizing
- Justifying
- Spiritualizing
- Denying
- Blame-shifting
- Ignoring / disregarding
- Gaslighting
- Raging

[1] WHAT IS EMOTIONAL ABUSE?

Rationalizing is explaining or justifying one's behavior, beliefs, or decisions in a way that makes them seem rational or logical, despite being harmful.

Minimizing downplays, dismisses, or invalidates the emotions, experiences, concerns, or autonomy of the victim.

Justifying is providing excuses, explanations, or rationalizations for the abusive behavior of the perpetrator.

Spiritualizing exploits spiritual beliefs, practices, or values in order to control, manipulate, or justify their abusive behavior.

Denying is a refusal or dismissal of the experiences, feelings, or needs of the victim by the abuser.

Blame-shifting deflects responsibility for harmful actions or behavior and places the blame onto the victim.

Disregarding or ignoring is dismissing the needs, emotions, boundaries, and well-being of the victim by the abuser.

Gaslighting undermines another person's perception of reality, memory, or sanity. The term seems to come from the 1938 British play *Gas Light* by Patrick Hamilton, which portrays a "seemingly genteel husband using lies and manipulation to isolate his heiress wife and persuade her that she is mentally unwell so that he can steal from her" by secretly dimming and brightening indoor gas-powered lights while insisting his wife is imagining things, leading her to think she is going insane.)

Raging is the use of derogatory language, insults, or verbal attacks by one partner towards the other, aimed at demeaning, belittling, or humiliating them.

(See the back of this book for more on these terms.)

The end result of the abuser using these tactics and behaviors is that the person being harmed feels crazy or as if they are losing their mind. Their confidence in their own perception of reality is undermined. They lose confidence in themselves and in their abilities as a person. They have more internal stress, as well as feel trapped and exhausted.

These are not exhaustive definitions, and there are many nuances and contexts that are important, but I want to caution you to avoid comparing your situation to others.

Freedom can never be obtained from comparison.

What I Hear . . .

The number one issue I repeatedly hear from emotionally abused women is, "I feel crazy." Here's a common scenario: You bring up a specific issue with your partner,[3] but you never arrive at a resolution. The other person always finds a way out of being accountable. You end up feeling like you're on a merry-go-round of discussions, or what I call "looping

[1] WHAT IS EMOTIONAL ABUSE?

arguments." You feel like you're walking on eggshells, afraid to bring anything up because you just go round and round, always ending up in the same bad place over and over and over again.

The other person takes *no* responsibility, leaving you with *all* the responsibility. They have the type of responsibility I call Teflon. Nothing sticks to them. You, on the other hand, are like Velcro. *Everything* becomes your responsibility.

This tiresome example is a key component for understanding emotional abuse:

> *Being stuck on an emotional merry-go-round will wear you out internally and overwhelm you.*

Some Reasons for the "Crazy"

Oftentimes, the abuser has a very good public image. Everyone outside of the relationship thinks they are a person of good character—untouchable. Behind closed doors, they're *not* so great. And no one knows this but you. The abuser has such a good reputation that when you finally work up the courage to share something with someone, you appear crazy, and many make you out to be a liar.

Have you ever been on the receiving end of one of these conversations?

- "Oh, Nancy. Are you sure? He's such a nice guy."
- "I have a hard time believing that, Carol. I have so much respect for your husband."
- "But I've watched him coach Timmy's soccer team, and he's so good with the kids."
- "Shirley, but he's done so much for this community."
- "Beth! How can you say that? He's your husband and our pastor!"

One indication of emotional abuse is that the abuser is one person in public, yet you experience another person in private. How can this abusive person be kind, compassionate, loving, and selfless in public and then be completely different when you're alone?

One indication of emotional abuse is that the abuser is one person in public, yet you experience another person in private.

Denial is when *an emotional abuser believes their own lies.* The Teflon partner turns everything back on you even when they are responsible. They believe the lie that any problem that arises is your fault. They make you believe that you're responsible for everything negative. *They fully believe it.* That's

[1] WHAT IS EMOTIONAL ABUSE?

why they can look you dead in the eye and lie to you. You feel crazy because every question you ask and every thought or instinct you have is denied, rationalized, minimized, justified, or spiritualized.

DOCUMENT

The first step to freedom is to identify and document all that you are feeling and experiencing. Doing so will help you clearly understand that what you are identifying is indeed emotional abuse.

A word of caution: As you're going through this process, don't talk to merely anyone who will listen about what you're going through. The average person in your circle of friends is not likely to have endured emotional abuse. As a result, their lack of firsthand experience will cause more confusion for you. It might even put people who love your spouse on the defense because of their own denial. Be careful about whom you talk to.

The first "person" you should talk to is a blank sheet of paper where you can write honestly about what you're feeling. Make sure what you write is not discoverable. Buy a lockbox and bury it in the backyard. Do whatever you have to do to maintain privacy. If you're not certain that your document is going to be safe, then you won't be honest. You're already afraid of being honest. That's why you're reading this book. You believe you're in an emotionally abusive relationship that makes you feel insecure and uncertain about who you are. So write, write, write. You'll learn about and discover who you are as you go. There are digital apps you can download for notes and journals that have passwords, which might feel safer to you than writing on paper.

The Church and Emotional Abuse

Unfortunately, in my experience, emotional abuse within the church is common. People in that environment appear to be spiritual and use their Bible, their position in the community, and their authority, as a way to keep you in a very difficult place. Because they're such shining examples of a "good Christian," they're able to rally other people around them to make you appear crazy. But I'm here to tell you that you're not. They might say things like, "You're just not a submissive enough wife," or "If you would just cook better meals, he'd be kinder," or "If you'd have more sex with him, everything would get better." *But these statements are all lies!*

Being submissive, cooking better meals, and having more sex doesn't work when you live with an abuser. *With all the effort you have already put in, your relationship should be out of this world!* But it isn't, it's destroying your soul. Here's the truth: The reason why abusers abuse has nothing to do with their partner.

The reason why abusers abuse has nothing to do with their partner.

[1] WHAT IS EMOTIONAL ABUSE?

If you give an abuser an inch, they'll take a mile. Abusers don't change because you do more for them. That's *not* how they change. In fact, they rarely change under any circumstances.

> *Abusers don't change because you do more for them.*

Church culture has made countless devastating mistakes. Situations involving emotional abuse have been frequently mishandled, and it has redefined the value of a "church" community for many women as a result. (I could write another book about that alone.) If you tell someone in the church about the abuse and they don't believe you, *then don't talk to them.* Unfortunately, the church is often one of the worst places you can go for help.

I'm saying this as a guy who planted a church and pastored it for years. I've talked to thousands of people in at least a hundred churches, and it's a fact: The church, because of its theological views, deems men to be more valuable than women. Many churches would not admit this openly, but the thinking and behavior are still there. There is a common theology that men always get the last say—husbands often have the last say in any issue. This creates and feeds a factory for narcissistic men and abused women.

DEATH OF A THOUSAND CUTS

> *There is a common theology that men always get the last say ... This creates and feeds a factory for narcissistic men and abused women.*

This also creates a culture in which marriage is idolized—the idea that because marriage is sacred it *must* be maintained *no matter what.* Nothing, not even abuse, should absolve a marriage. This is bad theology that doesn't, as a rule, believe the woman who is being abused.[4]

To put it plainly: If you tell your pastor about the abuse and he doesn't believe you, *then don't go back.* You'll only get harmed again if you do. If your pastor focuses on your need to forgive your husband rather than your husband's need to treat you and your family in a healthy way, *don't go back.* You must break free from this kind of faith community in order to find freedom from abuse.

You will encounter physical symptoms with emotional abuse. Living under chronic emotional stress will wear you out physically. Some physical results related to chronic stress are fibromyalgia, energy depletion, hair loss, and chronic fatigue. Adrenal fatigue—inadequate amounts of natural hormones—is also common to those in abusive relationships because you're always on guard. Let me give you a way to understand this better: Imagine starting up your car, leaving it in Park, and pushing the accelerator to the floor. What would happen? Do you think it's going to shorten the engine life? Of course! It's

[1] WHAT IS EMOTIONAL ABUSE?

guaranteed, even if it survives the hour, the engine life *will* be shortened. Whether you feel it or not, whether or not you're even conscious of it, this is a good picture of what's being done to you.

You are not designed to run at the red line. You can't *always* be on your guard *all* of the time. When you live like that, you're going to be emotionally and physically affected. I hear about the results of the constant stress from women all the time—the difficulty sleeping, feelings of overwhelm, being reactive, and having no patience. This is because all of your "internal space" is being used up to avoid getting harmed. You are constantly trying to figure out how to avoid the next attack, constantly trying to anticipate what they're going to do next.

> *You are constantly trying to figure out how to avoid the next attack, constantly trying to anticipate what they're going to do next.*

The reason it's important to document your feelings is so you can clearly understand them. Remember, your abuser is going to say that you're too sensitive, you're overreacting, or imply that you're defective in some way. Take a moment's pause and tell yourself to let their comments roll off you. Their destructive words are lies, and their abuse is causing you to feel overwhelmed and stressed out.

DEATH OF A THOUSAND CUTS

Emotional abuse is hard to define because it's layered and nuanced. It can take numerous interactions with the abuser for you to begin reacting from a place of hypervigilance and constant stress. If a woman comes into my office with a black eye, I immediately think, *We know what's going on here. She's been harmed. Let's rally the troops and help her!* Right?

However, when a woman comes into my office and she appears physically uninjured, it's not as easy to spot the problem right away. Emotionally abused women are experts at looking good. They are trained to pretend, to be survivors, to appear composed, and to not tell anybody the dark happenings behind closed doors. After all, that's what they're supposed to do, right? Well, that's what her abuser has told her, or even threatened. "Honey, you need to look good. Pull yourself together and smile. Always smile." Meanwhile, she is bleeding to death from a thousand internal cuts on the inside.

This is why abuse is so hard to define. A woman in an emotionally abusive relationship is dying the death of a thousand cuts. It's not one thing that will eventually take the life from her, it's a thousand things all put together. To look at just one cut out of a thousand, you'd think, *Ah, that's not too big of a deal. He was just a little bit upset and said something mean.* However, when you're talking about a consistent pattern occurring over a long period of time, it builds up. The bottom line is this: It takes somebody who actually understands the abuse to help you.

[1] WHAT IS EMOTIONAL ABUSE?

> *A woman in an emotionally abusive relationship is dying the death of a thousand cuts. It's not one thing that will eventually take the life from her, it's a thousand things all put together.*

There's a big difference between being emotionally abused and being in a difficult relationship. *Every* relationship is difficult. If you don't have any difficulties, then you can't have true intimacy. [5] A healthy, intimate relationship requires emotional vulnerability, but emotional and physical abuse are the things that kill vulnerability. As a result, vulnerability is off the table for these partnerships. It cannot be one-sided either. It must be mutual. When a woman walks into my office and describes one disastrous event, it's hard for me to determine if it's emotional abuse or simply a difficult relationship.

Difficult is different than *destructive*. In an emotionally abusive relationship, you're dealing with the systematic destruction of a soul—which is a classic pattern of abusive behavior.

> *Difficult is different than destructive. In an emotionally abusive relationship, you're dealing with the systematic destruction of your soul.*

DEATH OF A THOUSAND CUTS

You have probably met guys who say they love you and who you believe to be godly men. But then you notice them begin to systematically destroy your soul. *I'm telling you that God would never validate anyone being systematically destroyed.* I want to help you understand that being systematically destroyed is what's happening to you if you're in an emotionally abusive relationship.

[2]

WHAT IS SPIRITUAL ABUSE?

SPIRITUAL ABUSE SEEMS like an oxymoron, doesn't it? How could something be spiritual *and* be abusive? Unfortunately, this duo is a very common reality. If you're in an emotionally abusive relationship and you and your spouse are Christians, I can almost guarantee that you are being spiritually abused too. I'm going to present some principles I believe about God that might enlighten your view on the spiritual life.

God never devalues life. He is the author of life.

DEATH OF A THOUSAND CUTS

God never devalues life.
He is the author of life.

We often say, "God is love," right?[6] But do you always experience love? I don't. Sometimes I get upset and ask God, "Where are You? If You are love, then what are You doing? Why don't I see justice? Why aren't You changing things?" I get mad and hurt and want things to be different, but they don't change. I shake my head and think, *God, what are You doing?*

One of the things that helped me begin to understand the nature of God and His love was the birth of my first child. As a physically and emotionally abused person, I never got to experience and know what love truly was. What I understood love to be wasn't actually love at all, it was abuse and control.

When my first baby was born, I instantly connected with him. As both of us grew, the connection deepened, and I experienced love I didn't even know existed. I cared for my child in a way I had never even conceived of. Personally, I didn't know I was capable of being nurturing and offering unconditional love. As a result, I became very afraid that I might lose him because for the first time in my life, I valued *someone* above myself.

I'll tell you a funny story: After our first child was born, I told my (then) wife, "We can't have any more kids."

She looked at me, confused, and replied, "What do you mean? Why?"

[2] WHAT IS SPIRITUAL ABUSE?

I answered, "Because I can't love anyone else the way I love him. I don't think I have enough love. I didn't know I had *this* love. There's no way I'd be able to love someone else."

Guess what? I've spent my life loving that son *and* the son who came after him equally. I discovered I could love two kids just as much as I loved one. This profound, inconceivable love was revealed to me through the love I have for my sons. There's nothing they can do to stop me from loving them. I'm never going to turn from them, no matter what.

When we talk about God in church, we talk about Him being a loving Father. But what is a loving Father? What does that even look like? After I became a father, I realized God was telling me He's *my* Father, but I had never known what a loving father was. All I knew was how to survive my father. There was no love, only dodging his abuse and placating him if I could. So when God, who declared He was my Father, said He is love, it never computed within my soul. It may sound weird, but I really could not fathom *father* equaling *love*.

God loves me the way I love my sons, and even more. I couldn't imagine that kind of love when I held my newborn son, and I still have a hard time imagining that kind of love now. How about you? What's God going to say to you when you fail? "You stupid, good-for-nothing daughter. I can't believe it! I died on the cross for you, and you're messing up ... again! When are you going to get your life together?" No, He would never say that, nor would He want you to believe those things about yourself. God is loving, warmhearted, and welcoming: "Honey, I'm here. Let Me clean that wound. Let Me be with you."

One of the main things about God that we need to focus on is what I like to call His "withness." We talk about it at Christmas every year. Jesus is called Emmanuel, which means "God with us," but what does that *really* mean to us in our everyday lives? When Jesus came to Earth, He wasn't here to make sure people *believed* the right things. He wasn't here to make sure they *did* the right things. He came to *be with* us. Just like I want to *be with* my kids. Whether they're having joyful mountaintop experiences or they are in the valley, destroyed by their pain, I want to *be with* them, not judge them for where they are. God, in the same way, wants to *be with* you.

One of the main things about God that we need to focus on is His "withness."

When you are in the throes of spiritual abuse, your abuser will tell you what *should* happen and *how* it should happen. You are told to be submissive, to "Do as I say" without question. If it doesn't happen the way the abuser says it should, then you're labeled as bad or wrong. Many churches will tell you that this is God's design. But God's design isn't to shame and take the blame without question. Yes, sometimes we get things wrong, but that does not mean our character should be devalued. When I correct my child, it's never punitive. I'm not going to harm him because he didn't follow the rules. I treat him with

[2] WHAT IS SPIRITUAL ABUSE?

care. The consequences might not be pleasant, but I'm trying to lovingly move him to a better place.

A healthy spiritual life is supposed to lead us into freedom, not into being controlled and harmed.

> *A healthy spiritual life is supposed to lead us into freedom, not into being controlled and harmed.*

God is a far better parent than you or I could ever be. If someone is using the Bible to twist spiritual "language" to suit their desires in order to punish you, make you feel bad, manipulate you, or get you to do what they want, that's an abuse of spiritual life. Don't let anyone abuse you spiritually. Trust me, there are those who will try, if they feel they have the right, to control your behaviors and thoughts. Unfortunately, the church has made an idol of marriage, at least from my experience.

Being involved in the church *and* being in an abusive relationship is rarely a healthy combination. Saving the marriage becomes the number one goal for those who feel they have a say in your decisions, such as a pastor, church members, elders, and friends. Staying married instead of creating a safe and healthy marriage environment for both people is of greater importance than acknowledging the abuse and allowing the abused person an exit plan.

DEATH OF A THOUSAND CUTS

MARRIAGE AS AN IDOL

Let's say you sit down with a pastor to talk about the difficulties in your marriage. But before you even sit down, the pastor probably has an agenda—to keep your marriage together at all costs. The underlining reason why pastors have this agenda is because of their theological belief that "God hates divorce." While I once gave that same advice, I have realized over time this is not what God is communicating to His people in regards to divorce. In fact, God introduced divorce as a way to protect people from the harm of a spouse.

I was a part of one of those churches that believed there was nothing—*nothing*—more important than keeping a marriage together … and that men always have the last say.

Another part of the pastor's agenda is that you have to agree with them. Here's what I mean by that: Many churches have become a place where conformity of belief is important. When the pastor is sitting with you, it is unconsciously implied that you must agree with his frame of reference about what the Bible says. If your pastor is doing that, he has idolized marriage. No judgment on that pastor, but don't engage with him about your marriage ordeals. Whether he knows it or not, you are being spiritually abused *by him*. This combination—keeping the marriage together at all costs and having to agree with the pastor—keeps him from being able to hear the issues, difficulties, and problems you are dealing with.

Some women I have counseled believe they can change the pastor's mind. If they can only talk to him and get him to see

[2] WHAT IS SPIRITUAL ABUSE?

the reality of the abuse they are enduring, then surely he would understand why she wants to leave. But in my experience, that is a fool's errand. You are almost certainly not going to change your pastor's mind. Don't expend your energy talking to your pastor if he tells you to just forgive your husband and keep the marriage together. It is more important to spend your energy identifying the spiritual abuse and then navigating around it.

The combination of these two—keeping the marriage together at all costs and having to agree with the pastor—keeps him from being able to hear the issues, difficulties, and problems you are dealing with.

> *The combination of these two*
> *—keeping the marriage together at all costs*
> *and having to agree with the pastor—*
> *keeps him from being able to hear*
> *the issues, difficulties, and problems*
> *you are dealing with.*

There's a truth about the church that's hard to hear. The bottom line of modern Christianity all boils down to the *conformity of belief.* That means it's no longer about the love of God, it's about you having the "right" theology. It's about how you fit in to church culture. Ask yourself: How many people go to church to be honest? In the general church culture, it's not acceptable. You're not allowed to freely be the person God created. You can't be yourself and walk through those church doors *as you are*. This forced personal repression is also a form of abuse and is the opposite of the example Jesus set for us.

Time and time again, we see in the Bible that Jesus is with people right in the middle of their mess. He never kicked them to the curb, berated them, or said, "When are you going to clean up this mess? When are you going to do something about your mistakes?" In fact, what He modeled was one way to "clean up the mess." Jesus' care is what transformed the people around Him. It wasn't just because He gave them the truth. He truly *cared* for people. Pain is what lets us know there is a problem, but care is what allows us to overcome it. Saying, "I'm right and you're wrong" is a phrase that I believe is the undergirding for all spiritual abuse. The church has made a huge mess of many things by being arrogantly "right" about things they have no business judging. Jesus doesn't look at you and say, "I'm right and you're wrong!" He *cares* for you.

Pain is what lets us know there is a problem, but care is what allows us to overcome it.

When it comes right down to it, if someone uses their interpretation of the Bible to devalue you, to judge your situation, or to give biased advice on how you're supposed to "fix it," then you are experiencing spiritual abuse. My advice is to remove yourself from that person socially and refrain from sharing anything else.

[2] WHAT IS SPIRITUAL ABUSE?

Jane's husband, Bill, is on the worship team at church, attends a men's Bible study, faithfully tithes, and helps out in the community when needed. Everyone in the church loves Bill. However, at home Bill is controlling, won't let Jane make her own decisions, forces her to have sex, and uses the Bible to justify his sexual aggression. Bill controls the people Jane can talk to, and he rages at her and calls her demeaning names when he feels she's not doing what he wants. Bill also controls the money and tells Jane that she is not a Proverbs 31[7] wife unless she stays within his unreasonable financial rules. He then goes back to church, leads worship, and is seen as a very caring Christian man.

"Jane" is a real woman I have worked with. While her name has been changed, this is a real scenario. I could give you one hundred more examples of marriages where the husband feels it's his right to manipulate, control, and take away a wife's freedoms while proclaiming it to be "God's will."

Another commonality among spiritually abused women is sometimes the church might see her husband as someone who needs to behave better, and she should wait for his transformation. So she goes home and (feeling a tiny bit understood by some people) sets boundaries that are strong enough to cause her abuser a little pain. He'll most always have an epiphany (albeit a false one). He'll start reading the Bible in front of her and become more involved at church (or begin going). He might try to win points and buddy up to the pastor. Everyone at church thinks it's a miracle! He seems to be changing, even begins therapy and starts working on himself.

DEATH OF A THOUSAND CUTS

He might start using counseling terms, to the disgust of his wife, who knows it's all smoke and mirrors. The wife might hear him say, "I'm becoming the man and the father you've always wanted me to be." Other people echo his "promise" back to her, glad they "don't have to do anything" or intervene because maybe the wife was being a little too demanding. Maybe she was overreacting, or simply bossing him around. Some even look at the abuser as the put-upon spouse who has to jump through hoops in order to please his wife.

Meanwhile, what he's really doing is spiritually abusing her, so she stops enforcing the boundaries.

The point I hope you understand is that *spiritual abuse often increases when boundaries are set.* If someone changes because you set a boundary, they are not changing from an internal motive. Authentic transformation must be measured over time and paired with consistent behavioral transformation. A false or forced epiphany does not initiate a heartfelt transformation. A false epiphany typically initiates a fear-based, short-term reaction that only appears to be a true transformation.

Spiritual abuse often increases when boundaries are set.

Revelation minus transformation equates to manipulation. An abuser's change might seem like an improvement, but 99 percent of the time, the abuser has a *false* epiphany. *False* action always follows a false epiphany.

[2] WHAT IS SPIRITUAL ABUSE?

Revelation minus transformation equates to manipulation… False action always follows a false epiphany.

DEATH OF A THOUSAND CUTS

[3]

CODEPENDENCY IS EXTERNAL DEPENDANCE

WHAT IS CODEPENDENCY? It depends on who you ask. There's a lot of information out there, and many in the psychology field have varying definitions. My definition is different from most that you'll read. I define codependence as "external dependence," which is the process of your soul and *your value as a person* becoming dependent on external realities. External dependance is defined as someone who derives their value as a human being based on whether other people approve of them or not. Value comes from outside sources instead of being generated from within one's self.

You lose internal value when you depend upon the external. It's as if your value is bleeding out into your circumstances. A dependence on the external motivates you to be overly concerned about what others think of you, your circumstances, and how those circumstances will be resolved.

How External Dependance Mixes with Emotional Abuse

External dependance is a toxic mix when paired with emotional abuse. If you believe that it's your job to make someone else happy, then your abuser is going to use that as leverage to control you. When you believe your job is to make other people happy, you are easily abused. But your abuser's well-being is *not* your responsibility. It doesn't matter what the abuser thinks or feels. It is your right to *not* be responsible for someone else's well-being. It is healthy for you to detach from the abuser's problems and instead focus on yourself.

---

*If you believe it's your job
to make someone else happy,
then your abuser is going to use that
as leverage to control you.*

Many Christians, pastors, and church groups have instilled the message that women are responsible for the well-being of their husbands. It has become a theological undergirding that is simply not true. One falsehood I've heard many times is that you'll win your husband over with your winsome behavior.

[3] CODEPENDENCY IS EXTERNAL DEPENDANCE

Those women, and you may be one of them, are also being told they are responsible for the happiness, success, and salvation of their husbands. But Jesus is the one in charge of that, not a spouse.

In Christian circles, pressure is mainly placed upon the women to become externally dependent. In other words, their value is predicated on whether or not someone else is happy or healthy. But that's *not* how it works.

THE ORIGIN OF EXTERNAL DEPENDENCE

Maybe you grew up in a home where the family pathology indicated that it was the woman's job to make other people happy. You may have watched your mom take care of your dad. You saw that he was unkind to your mom, but she never said or did anything to stand up for herself. No one actually said that was how you should live. But kids don't do what their parents say, they *do* what their parents *do*. Kids pick things up by osmosis, forming the patterns for their adult life. You may have a family pathology that was embedded in you at such an early age that you believe it is how you were wired. In actuality, you were trained by your parents to adopt certain behaviors and beliefs.

One of the main consequences of external dependence is that you lose yourself, and your true essence vanishes or becomes vacant. That means you feel little joy and contentment in everyday life. Your identity becomes hijacked because you have traded in your self-worth for outside approval. You feel relief when you satisfy someone else's standards. This is a no-win proposition for the person who is externally dependent.

One of the main consequences to external dependance is that you lose yourself.

BENEFITS OF *NOT* BEING EXTERNALLY DEPENDENT

The positive consequence of getting out of external dependence is that you become a whole person. You recognize yourself as the legitimate and viable human you always were. That has never been in question. It's just that you didn't believe it. This is why you must get out of relationships that set you up to be the savior, the doormat, the cause of all evil, or the reason for *all* of the problems. Getting out of those types of relationships is paramount to recovering from external dependance.

As a culture, we view the act of leaving a relationship as negative, even if it's obvious the relationship is unhealthy. Sometimes those unhealthy relationships are with our family members. Staying in unhealthy relationships only solidifies the fact that you will end up in an abusive relationship.

[3] CODEPENDENCY IS EXTERNAL DEPENDANCE

Here are two rules that will help you discern when your relationship has become externally dependent:

> Rule #1: No crazy allowed.
>
> Rule #2: I decide what's crazy.

When someone is externally dependent, they never have the right to make the decision about what is defined as crazy. As somebody who has been externally dependent, the greatest victory I ever had was to stop putting myself in that position and take back authority over my own choices. One of the things that happens when we live in abusive relationships is that we lose our ability to choose because we fear the consequences of exerting our free will.

> *One of the things that happens when we live in abusive relationships is that we lose our ability to choose.*

As a kid, I couldn't choose what I wanted. My only option was to comply in order to keep the abuse from occurring, though complying didn't always keep me from abuse, either. I didn't get to choose what I wanted to do or how I would spend the day. My only job was to comply with my parents' demands and expectations. As I got older and began my recovery journey, I realized *I have choices*. But then I started to feel like I was "bad" if I took the reins of my life and made a choice. This kind of thinking kept me stuck in other people's worlds, doing *what* they wanted and doing it *how* they wanted.

Other people will get upset when you start to make choices for yourself. These people will want you to go back to your role of making them happy. The family pathology is usually the most determined at keeping you in your role. This means you're going to have to go through a process of losing some relationships. Yes, you might have to pull away from certain family relationships in order to leave external dependence.

It's impossible to recover from external dependence and keep all of your relationships because the people within those relationships don't want you to change. They want you to keep feeding their narcissism. They want you to keep being *their* codependent to keep *their* lives working so they won't have to deal with *their own* stuff. I mean, someone has to be the scapegoat.

But when you break free of external dependence, you can return to the valuable life God created you to have. Your value is intrinsic and beautiful. Embracing *God's value of you* is how you're going to overcome the trap of external dependence.

---

*Embracing God's value of you is how
you're going to overcome the trap
of external dependence.*

---

[4]

CLEARING & CREATING INTERNAL STRENGTH

I'VE WORKED WITH many people, particularly women, who have been in emotionally abusive relationships. They live in an emotionally dangerous environment. In order to begin healing from the emotional pain, there are some very important concepts about your core beliefs that need to be present. To begin the process of healing, you'll need to have the courage to set boundaries. But in order to do that, you're going to have to develop your internal strength, which is built upon your core beliefs.

DEATH OF A THOUSAND CUTS

> *To begin the process of healing, you'll need to have the courage to set boundaries. But to do that, you're going to have to develop your internal strength.*

You may think it's not possible to change your core beliefs, but I'm here to tell you it is. The concepts I'm going to talk about in this chapter are the foundation of your transformational power. I'm not going to focus on the other person—the abuser—who is harming you. I'm going to focus on *you*. Why? Because developing your strength and hope on an internal level is imperative for you to be able to move through the abuse in a healthy way so you can get to a place of freedom.

CORE CONCEPTS FOR TRANSFORMATIONAL POWER

What I have observed and experienced and, consequently, believe is that everyone has a limited amount of space for emotional content.

> *Everyone has a limited amount of space for emotional content.*

[4] CLEARING & CREATING INTERNAL STRENGTH

Let's say you have your very best day planned out. You're going to engage in your favorite activity with your favorite people in beautiful weather. You can't wait! It's going to be awesome! Then, on your very best day, something happens. A guy in the car in front of you cuts you off. Your kid wakes up in a bad mood. Your spouse says something harmful. Or out of nowhere a negative memory shows up you didn't want to replay.

Imagine for a moment that we each have an "internal box" where we each have a limited amount of space available to hold emotional content. In my experience, we each have a *different* limit, but we each have a limit. The internal box is filled up over time by events we see as harmful to us. Regardless of how big of an event it is (or isn't), the key is that *we feel it as harmful*. Let's call it *negative emotional input*. This content is usually something we have no control over, the harmful actions of others.

For example, in my childhood there was a lot of harm, and *by the time I was a teen my internal box was full*. So moving forward, any normal life event could be perceived as having negative emotional content. I would then have a "level 8" reaction to a "level 2" event *because I was already full*. This all lies just beneath our conscious awareness until we start to take the time to document, which makes us more conscious and makes connections between what happened to us and our reactions. We start to understand.

Even on your very best day, you have *negative* emotional input. If you have negative emotional input and your "internal box" is already full, what's going to happen? Generally, *something has to go out*. Something has to leave. What does this process look like for you? What do you do? What is your reaction? How do you handle the negative input?

As we just saw, reactions to negative emotional inputs often happen subconsciously, so you may not have an awareness of how you respond. Yet it is important to become aware of what's happening inside you when encountering a negative emotional input. Some people use substances, use people, or use some other kind of distraction. My old response to negative input was to isolate myself. Isolation was one of my favorite reactions. Another old response for me was sinking into depression. Or I would use religion to boost my ego. I would become "good" or do good things as a way to distract myself from the pain. Try to become aware of how you respond.

If you are full—and I'm assuming you are because you're in an abusive relationship—what filled you up? Did your childhood fill you up? Maybe you were already full when you met your abuser. Your childhood experiences may have been the underlying reasons you were lured into your current abusive relationship. *We are drawn to what we know, even if it is harmful to our body and soul.* If a chaotic and abusive childhood was your normal, then your current abusive relationship feels "good enough." At least this way, you will know what to expect. Unfortunately, this mindset also makes you less likely to see the red flags surfacing in someone's behavior. Many deny these red flags even exist.

[4] CLEARING & CREATING INTERNAL STRENGTH

The message of toxic shame says, *You don't matter. You're defective. You're less-than. You're not worth the skin you're living in. There's something wrong with you.* Everyone who has a full internal world also has some version of this message in their heart and soul. Now add a relationship with someone who tells you these negative things on a regular basis, *whether outright or implied*.

Communication through implication is much worse than being told outright. I mean, how can you challenge your abuser based on an implication? They didn't really say anything, they just implied it. One of the most powerful ways an abuser implies things about you is by *disregarding* you. For instance, when they walk into the room, they don't acknowledge you. They don't offer a friendly greeting. They act as if they don't see you or notice you are there.

Imagine a husband who goes to the kitchen for something but never offers to get anything for his wife. People outside the home never see this. At church, he is kind and helpful to everyone. But at home the wife is constantly disregarded by her supposedly wonderful husband.

Another common tactic abusers use to foster toxic shame is through *gaslighting*. This is the husband who says, "I never said that. You heard it wrong." This implies you are wrong. You're not good enough. You don't matter. But the fact is, you didn't hear it wrong, *he did* say that, and you do matter.

These are just two of the numerous ways abusers can imply that you don't matter. Disregard, in particular, is a profound way that someone can say "You don't matter." Disregard is most painful when it comes from the person who says they love you because you end up thinking, *I just have to try harder.*

What if you believe the message that says, *I don't matter?* You might engage one of your coping mechanisms, such as isolation, using a substance, using people, or clinging to religion, which is filtered through the "I don't matter" message. Instead of addition, you now have multiplication! You're in trouble because you believe you're the problem. You feel like there's no way out because your behavior is proving the message!

Hold a mirror up to your internal world. Can you see engines for shame in your life? Do you understand how this is happening within you? If you're in an emotionally abusive relationship, you have someone who is pouring gasoline on the "I don't matter" message because they *want* you to be harmed. They don't want you feeling well.

How do we erase some of what's in your internal box? First, let's talk about what's in there. What life experiences have filled your internal world? This explains why your box is full. Injustice, in particular, is an unfair and unwanted violation and damages your life. If you're in an emotionally abusive relationship, you've experienced a lot of injustice. Is it possible your injustice started before the relationship you're in now? More often than not, that's the case.

One common denominator among every human being is injustice. No one escapes. Everyone is impacted by injustice.

[4] CLEARING & CREATING INTERNAL STRENGTH

*One common denominator
among every human being is injustice.
No one escapes.
Everyone is impacted by injustice.*

We often ask ourselves, "Why is this happening to me?" I don't know the answers to these questions, but I do know that everyone has experienced injustice, and some more than others. But the issue isn't whether or not you've experienced injustice. The health of your life really has more to do with what *you do* with the injustice. How you handle it will be the determining factor in whether you have a healthy or unhealthy life. If you're in an emotionally abusive relationship, what you're being told, taught, and pressured to do is:

- Ignore
- Rationalize
- Minimize
- Justify
- Deny
- Take the blame

These responses are what fill up your box. They then make you so emotionally weak that you feel unable and unequipped to fight. I want to help you build the strength you need to start fighting back, because you're going to have to fight. I wish there was an easy way to get to that place, or a magic pill that could make it all go away, but fighting for yourself will be a real challenge.

When you suffer injustice, you must decide what you're going to do with that injustice. First, you must start documenting it.

> *When you suffer injustice, you must decide what you're going to do with that injustice. First, you must start documenting it.*

It's important to understand that injustice can be real or perceived. Here's what I mean: My father abused me. This was a real injustice. On a totally different day, perhaps years later, I see some guy and I think, *That guy doesn't like me*. I've never met the guy, but I can just tell by the look on his face: *That guy doesn't like me, just like my dad.* This is perceived injustice. You may have a lot of perceived injustice too. It doesn't matter whether it's real or perceived. Once you feel the injustice, it's yours and it's going to affect you.

There's something else about injustice. It hurts. On the surface, what we reveal or what we allow others to see is anger. Anger is what reaches the surface, but underneath the anger is injustice. In an emotionally abusive relationship, are you allowed to be angry? No, not according to your abuser! Only your spouse is *allowed* to be angry. Only the person abusing you

[4] CLEARING & CREATING INTERNAL STRENGTH

is allowed to be angry. Was that what happened to you as a child? Were you not allowed to express your feelings? Were you supposed to be appropriate, good, please people, and not get upset?

As you examine the things in your box, be sure to document them. If you doubt that something is in your box, write it down anyway. You may have been programmed to suppress events that took place or suppress your feelings about those events. Emotionally abused individuals are often programmed to ignore all of what's in their box. If you ignore what's inside, you're never going to heal or have the strength to fight. Even if you are able to get out of your current relationship, you won't be able to heal. You have to heal from the injustice in order to reach a place where you can healthily connect with another person.

You have to fight the programming. You're programmed to suppress. You're programmed to ignore all of what's in your box. If you ignore it, then you're never going to heal.

> *You're programmed to ignore all of what's in your box. If you ignore it, you're never going to heal.*

I know you may not believe this, but anger is healthy. How do I know you may have trouble believing that statement? Because people are often told that anger is bad: "You should never be angry." It's worse for those in abusive relationships because anger is only bad when the victim is angry, but when the abuser is angry (who is usually a male), then anger is okay. This common belief about anger is totally unhealthy and allows abuse to thrive.

But hold on! There is such a thing as *healthy anger*.

Healthy Anger

What does healthy anger look like? If you are in a relationship with someone and they say something harmful to you, then you might say, "Ow! That hurt!" Is that appropriate? Yes, that is healthy, appropriate anger. In an abusive relationship, you're supposed to just take it, which is not appropriate or healthy.

Initially, you won't be able to go to your abuser and say, "Hey, that hurt me." You haven't found your internal strength yet. Finding that strength is still in its infancy. Remember, document your feelings in writing. Put them on paper. The process of documenting your feelings isn't going to happen quickly, and you're going to want to resist and avoid it. But you *have* to start documenting because when you do, you'll start to understand your situation clearly.

Document your feelings in writing.
You're going to start to understand
your situation clearly.

---

[4] CLEARING & CREATING INTERNAL STRENGTH

As you get clarity, you're going to get angry because you'll soon become aware of how much injustice you have been living with. The denial will fall away, and you'll start to *really* see. Step back a moment and think: *If your anger matched the injustice you've experienced, how angry would you be?* By answering this one question, you will be flooded with some of the biggest lightbulb moments of your life! "Oh my gosh! He's just like my dad!" or "I see a pattern! Every time he says, 'such and such,' I feel shameful and guilty!"

Clarity is what we're working toward, which will lead you to a place of internal strength. I'll share a story to illustrate what I'm talking about. Years ago, I worked in a treatment center and was contracted with a medical clinic and an insurance company to provide drug and alcohol services to people with dependency issues. One day, the doctor called me and said, "Hey, Pat. I need some help."

"Sure, man. What can I do?" I replied.

"I have a client who is sixteen years old, and I'm giving him more pain meds than I can justify. He has this non-specified gut pain. I believe the kid is in pain, but I've got him on so many meds. I don't know that adding more is going to help him. I've done every test known to man, but I can't find a cause for this kid's pain. Can you come in and talk to him? My goal is to get him to take less medicine. Maybe you can help with that?"

"Glad to do it. I'll come talk to the kid," I said.

DEATH OF A THOUSAND CUTS

When I started meeting with the boy, I knew it was going to take some time to develop rapport, but the kid was very amenable and open. He started coming down on his meds. One of the things I said to him was, "Look, we'll bring your medicine down, but if your pain goes up, then we'll increase the medicine again. If your pain continues to stay the same, we'll bring your medicine down and see if we can get rid of some of these side effects. Okay?"

After working with this kid for a period of time, I started to learn some things. I learned his father was in prison for murder, and his mom was remarried to a guy who was very abusive to her. I asked, "Hey, man, what's it like at home?"

He said, "My stepdad is mean to my mom."

This kid was about six-foot-two and big, but because of his illness he was weak and could barely function enough to make it through each day.

"How do you handle that?" I asked.

"Oh, I don't. If I had more energy, I'd probably beat the guy up," he responded.

In my mind and my gut, I was beginning to think this abusive man knew that if this kid was healthy, he would be in trouble. I also believed the stepdad was poisoning the kid's food to make him ill, and I told the doctor as much.

The doctor looked at me, shocked and confused, and said, "Doyle, you've been working in treatment too long. That's way out there. You should not be suggesting this or accusing someone of illegal activity. That's crazy! No way!"

[4] CLEARING & CREATING INTERNAL STRENGTH

"Well, I don't know, man. I'm going to explore it some more," I told him.

I kept asking the boy questions and found out during our next session that his stepdad did all the cooking. Red flags were waving wildly in my mind's eye. I knew something was wrong. I went back to the doctor and said, "Look, we have to test him for what can cause these symptoms."

Sure enough, this kid was being poisoned on a regular basis with just enough poison to keep him ill. The stepdad had done his research and knew what he was doing. It wasn't going to kill the kid, but it would make him chronically sick and in pain in order to keep him weak. When the doctor did the testing and found out what it was, we were able to finally get the kid the help he needed.

Now, that's a graphic illustration of what your injustice will do to you. It'll keep you so sick that you can't fight your abuser. But you need to fight your abuser! You need to develop your internal strength. You need to heal, not continue to avoid. As I said before, I want you to work toward *not* spending so much time on your abuser and start spending more time on yourself and what's going on inside *you*.

You're not going to heal everything. You're just going to take out a corner of your internal box. Yet, taking out only a corner is like creating a whole new life! Having that much space and freedom will be inconceivable at first. Document what's going on and be as honest as possible. That's where I want you to start. As you do, identify the behaviors that are linked to what you're feeling internally and become aware of them. If you don't have somebody in your life you can talk to, then talk to the paper. Doing this will move you from "I don't" to "I *do* matter."

If you have a good therapist or a good friend who understands emotional abuse who is connected to you, please talk to them because the more you can externalize this stuff, the clearer you'll become.

SECTION II:

FIND REAL HOPE

DEATH OF A THOUSAND CUTS

[5]

THE TRUTH ABOUT TRUST & HEALING

THERE ARE CERTAIN questions that I hear a lot:

How do I know if my spouse is changing?

How do I know if his repentance or change is real?

How do I know if I should trust him again?

Can you spot the subtext in these questions: Is there *real* repentance and change? All of these questions are valid and must be asked. Unfortunately, the common teaching you will hear at church, and what many women hear directly from their pastor, usually bypasses these questions and jumps straight to,

"Well, you should forgive him." Which, in essence, means you should reconcile, trust, and continue to have a relationship with your abuser.

However, reconciliation and trust are *not* the same as forgiveness and healing. They are separate realities.

---

*Reconciliation and trust
are not the same as forgiveness and healing.
They are separate realities.*

If you're healing from someone's harm or forgiving them, there is absolutely zero requirement that you reconcile or trust them. Reconciliation and trust are completely separate processes.

Going forward, as I discuss reconciliation and forgiveness, I'm going to use the terms *trust* and *healing* as a way to keep you clear on the objectives. My concern with the terms *reconciliation* and *forgiveness* are the unspoken spiritual implications that are packed into them. Now let's talk about rebuilding trust.

Reconciliation or Rebuilding Trust

What do you require in order to trust someone? Nothing. You're not required to trust anyone. Many Christians, including pastors and church leaders, bypass the process required for rebuilding trust by telling you that you must

[5] THE TRUTH ABOUT TRUST & HEALING

reconcile. In church language, reconciliation means trust. But remember that trust and reconciliation are not the same. Trust should never be on the table until the person who has been betrayed or harmed believes that the person who harmed them understands and has taken responsibility for their actions. You decide, not anyone else.

I see this scenario all the time: The person who harms you "apologizes" in a way that actually shifts the blame back to you: "I'm sorry, but if you hadn't done 'such and such,' I wouldn't have reacted that way." It sounds like an apology, but what they're really doing is blaming *you*.

WHAT IS YOUR GUT TELLING YOU?

Think about what your gut is telling you. I'm talking about your instincts, your internal voice, your spirit. For example, you're having a conversation with someone, and your instincts (your internal voice, your gut) are telling you the person is not being honest. But your brain says, *Uh, no. I can't say anything. I'll offend them. What if I'm wrong? What will they think of me?* One of the difficulties with trusting your gut is that it gives you information you cannot prove, you just know it. But trusting your gut is imperative to dealing with your abuser. All of the abuser's tactics are trying to get you to not trust your gut.

When your abuser is talking to you and your gut says one thing, but your head says another, what I'm asking you to document is what your gut says, *not* what your head says. This is how you can clarify what's going on inside of you, leading you to build internal strength. Being aware of what your gut is saying is the key to healing. I'm asking you to document what your gut is telling you as much as possible. When you document your instincts—aka your gut feelings—you are breaking the rule of suppression that the abuser has taught you.

Remember the questions at the beginning of the chapter? In order to know whether or not the change is real, you have to trust your gut, not your abuser's demands. Your trust has been broken. Just because he says "I'm sorry" doesn't mean you immediately trust him again. Here's an example. Someone asks a favor of you …

"Hey, can I borrow your car?"

"Okay. Sure, you can borrow my car," you respond.

That person borrows your car, wrecks it, and when they bring it back to you, they say, "Oh, I'm sorry. I got in a wreck with your car."

The next day, the same person comes to you and says, "Can I borrow your car again?"

"No!" you say, exasperated.

"Why?" they ask, as if nothing has happened.

"Well, because I can't trust you. You wrecked it," you answer logically.

"Hey, I said I was sorry," they counter, implying that you're expected to magically trust them. No! You get to decide who you trust and who you don't.

[5] THE TRUTH ABOUT TRUST & HEALING

In situations like these, you are often dealing with someone who is a blame shifter, rationalizer, minimizer, denier, gaslighter, or spiritualizer. In other words, it's *never* their fault, it's *always* yours. You are to blame for why they harmed you. Their argument is that they harmed you because you don't trust them. I want to empower you to *not* trust. You don't reconcile with someone until *you* are sure and confident the person who broke your trust is now trustworthy.

Over time, this repeatedly broken trust gets you to a place where you're completely closed down. You have maybe one molecule of softness left in your heart. It's natural and necessary to fiercely guard that last molecule. Guarding that molecule is the most loving thing you can do for yourself *and* the abuser. People at church, including your pastor, might say that you're "hardening your heart," but when you have been abused, being closed down is normal and healthy.

When Your Abuser Has an Epiphany

Let's say for the sake of argument that your abuser has an epiphany. He's on a new path, turning over a new leaf. He now understands and wants to love you the way *you* need to be loved. He suddenly wants to be the best husband ever … blah, blah, blah.

> *He suddenly wants to be the best husband ever … blah, blah, blah.*

DEATH OF A THOUSAND CUTS

I don't want to sound insensitive, but at this point his epiphany is only a string of meaningless words. You're closed down. So what should you do in the moment of this seemingly heartfelt profession? Should you open up and say, "Okay"?

No! That would be a tragic mistake.

Keeping your wall up during the abuser's epiphany is important. If your gut is telling you that it is genuine, you only take one brick down and see how they behave. *Trust is earned over time by trustworthy behavior.* As that trust is rebuilt, the lowering of your wall is connected to their trustworthy behavior as decided by you. Remember, trust is *your* decision.

One of the tricks of an abuser is you, as the victim, are *not* allowed to *not* trust. You're supposed to trust your abuser and keep allowing them to harm you. You are expected to keep taking the responsibility. The spiritually healthy thing to do is to protect yourself from their harm. Being devalued is never spiritually healthy. Telling your abuser that you're not going to allow him to harm you by saying, "I'm not going to trust you" is imperative. Trust is dependent on the other person's behavior, not yours.

Trust is dependent on the other person's behavior, not yours.

When your abuser says, "I'm sorry," let me suggest that you respond using the words from Missouri's motto. What do I mean by that? Missouri is the "show me" state. It doesn't

[5] THE TRUTH ABOUT TRUST & HEALING

matter what your abuser says, it's *all* about what they *do*. You should watch their behavior and then make a decision. That's a healthy way to move forward. Watching their behavior is the fulcrum for getting out of an emotionally abusive relationship. When you start to take their behavior seriously and establish boundaries, it will make the relationship very difficult for your abuser. He is going to employ even more manipulative tactics and come at you from different angles.

Being clear about the harm your abuser is doing, and your unwillingness to accept the harm, or to not trust your abuser until there's behavioral evidence that he has changed is actually healthy. Remember, real behavioral change has to be demonstrated consistently over an extended period of time. Trust is a choice you make based on proven behavioral changes that, *over time*, reveal the abuser is now trustworthy. Changed or new behavior is *not* an event. You're going to have to see that new behavior over time, so don't start lowering your protection at the first instance of a change in behavior. Be patient.

Changed Behavior and the Church

The concept of "changed behavior over time" seems to be something many people at church don't understand. Often, you will be told that you should "just forgive him." Translation: "Blindly trust him."

Don't do that!

Do not listen to anyone at church who tells you to blindly forgive your abuser. Whether they know it or not, they are inappropriately using God and the Bible to put you in harm's way. Trust is separate from forgiveness and healing. Trust is dependent on the abuser's changed behavior over time. You're not required to trust unless *you* decide to.

Forgiveness and Healing

What is forgiveness? What is healing? Is healing the same as saying, "What he did was okay"? Is forgiveness forgetting? How many times have you heard the phrase "forgive and forget"? I wish I could forget! My life would be *so* much easier if I could forget all of the abuse, but none of us are going to forget, so we can jettison that idea.

Just as forgiveness is not about forgetting, healing is not about avoidance. Healing is not between you and the offender. Healing is between *you* and the *Creator*. *You* go to the Creator and work through the pain of the betrayal, the pain of the harm, the loss of the relationship, and the loss of the trust. Forgiveness and healing are not an event, they are a process. Pastors and Christians like to talk about forgiveness as if it's an event. But that's not the case. It is *not* a one-time event.

---

*Forgiveness and healing are not an event,
they are a process.*

---

[5] THE TRUTH ABOUT TRUST & HEALING

Here's how it looked for me. As a kid in my twenties, I was driving down the road, minding my own business and having a good day, when suddenly a memory of being harmed by my dad popped into my head. I was instantly transported back to all of the pain and thoughts of revenge.

In that moment, what did I do? Did I clutch, grab, and hang on to that offense? Did I say, "Yeah, he's a wretched, horrible person!" Or did I begin to work through the process of forgiveness by looking at the pain honestly and saying, "You know what? That was awful and really sad. It really hurt me that my dad treated me that way."

Remember, forgiveness is a process. When I think of painful memories about my dad, I still acknowledge and recognize that the abuse was horrible. My dad was a very sick person. I needed help to let go of that pain so I could eventually live in the truth of saying, "I'm okay." I didn't ignore what hurt me, but I let the pain surface. I grieved the pain so that I could live my life in health.

I often hear a teaching in church that makes forgiveness out to be some magical thing where we act like the abuse didn't happen, as if I can forgive my dad without touching the pain. But if someone has harmed you, it *is* painful, and you must work through that pain in order to heal. Otherwise, what happens? You hold on to that pain, which makes you triggerable.

I'd like to use the analogy of abuse as an open wound on your soul. You've been "cut," and it's a gaping wound. If I poke your open wound, what's going to happen? You're probably going to have a very serious reaction. That's a *trigger*.

If the wound heals and becomes a scar and your scar is poked, there will be no reaction. You're never going to forget what happened, but you do have a scar to prove it and remember the injury.

Let's apply this concept to your internal wounds. All of these "cuts" are things people have said or done to you. If they are left as open wounds, avoided and unhealed, they become triggers. Triggers are not only harmful to others but harmful to you.

To continue the analogy, your abuser will jab a finger into your open wounds. Your reaction is probably going to be self-blame and shame. So it's important to stop and think about your wounds. Clarify who is responsible for them. For years, I thought I was responsible for the wounds my father inflicted. How could I forgive him when I was responsible? Clarifying that *my father* was responsible for my wounds ushered me into a new understanding. I discovered I needed to work through the pain and grief his wounding had caused. Working through pain, grief, and forgiveness was necessary; otherwise, the wounds would still have control over me. That's how healing works and why it's a process. As you work through the grief, you're being honest with yourself about what happened. As you become honest about the past, your open wound closes.

When somebody comes by and pokes you after you have healed, they won't get a reaction. Even better, now that your open wound has healed and there's a scar, the event that

[5] THE TRUTH ABOUT TRUST & HEALING

caused the scarring in the first place becomes a part of your strength. It's no longer your liability.

There is another reason not to leave your wounds open. As your wounds heal, you will have less reactivity to your abuser. Reactivity is one of the things an abuser is counting on. Because the abuser keeps harming you and poking your wounds, it's inevitable that you will react. The abuser will then blame you for being the abusive one because of your reactivity. But reacting when someone jabs their finger into your wound is normal. If someone jabs a healed wound—a scar—you are not going to react in the same way. That's why you have to clearly understand who is responsible for your wounds.

> *Because the abuser keeps harming you and poking your wounds, it's inevitable that you will react.*

PUTTING IT ALL TOGETHER

Forgiveness and healing are part of a process, not the main event, and they are separate from reconciliation and trust. Reconciliation and trust are *not* a requirement, no matter what you are told at church or by other Christians. Work through the process of forgiveness and healing one day at a time, and don't take responsibility for another person's behavior. Let *them* be responsible, and *do not* trust them until there's proof of real change.

"Real change?" You may say this with a skeptical tone. "How do I know if he has really changed?"

I get this question all the time, and here's my answer. You have to pay attention to your gut, to your instincts. If someone harms you and they recognize they harmed you and feel broken and sad about what they did, they will come to you without you having to say anything, look you in the eye, and say, "When I did *X* to you yesterday, I see how my behavior hurt you. I am sorry for this. I will show you through my actions by valuing you, not harming you."

Pay attention to your gut.

They will be specific about what they were apologizing for. If this is the case, your gut will give you some insight: *Oh, wow! They really get it. They really do know what they did.* Then you can safely lower your wall—just a little.

But if your abuser says, "I'm really sorry about what I did yesterday." They're not apologizing in a specific way. Your gut will provide your answer: *I don't believe him.*

You need to go with that.

Let your gut be the decider, not someone else's expectations. As you let your gut decide, you might even make a mistake. You might not let someone in when they're really sorry, yet you

[5] THE TRUTH ABOUT TRUST & HEALING

thought they weren't. But when it comes to trust, it's far better to be late to the party than early. The damage that can be done to you by trusting too soon is far greater than any damage that will happen if you wait to trust again.

Being late to the party of trust is actually another test of your abuser's repentance. Do they seem willing to change? Are they willing to take ownership for what they've done? If they're impatient with you not trusting them, that's a sign they're not really changing. When someone changes, they recognize, "I did this awful thing. It's going to take time, and I have to be patient. I'm going to experience pain because I caused the pain. I will do whatever it takes to make this relationship right."

False change, false apologies, and false repentance, these are what you get 99 percent of the time with abusers.

False change, false apologies and false repentance, these are what you get 99 percent of the time with abusers.

If instead the person who hurt you says, "This is taking forever! You *still* don't trust me? What do I have to do? I'm tired of waiting for *you* to grow up!" This person is irritated and impatient. That's a sign that their change is false. False change, false apologies, and false repentance is what you get 99 percent of the time with abusers.

THE FIRST STEP TO VALUING YOURSELF

When you trust your gut, it means that you're starting to value yourself. That's *very* exciting! Valuing yourself instead of the expectations of others is one of the main things that's going to get you through the healing process.

One of the questions I'm asked a lot is: Does forgiving the abuser make what they did okay? *No, never.* If someone harms you, it's *never* okay. This is another false understanding about forgiveness. Forgiveness takes time. It takes time to rebuild the trust. In order to do that, there needs to be separation in the relationship. If you don't separate and create distance so the trust can develop, you're going to have trouble. When someone harms you, distance is necessary in order to gain clarity. That's how it works. Your theology, your commitments, your friends at church, or your family may tell you, "You should just stay. It's no big deal. You're just being too sensitive." But you're being set up for deeper and more problematic harm.

When someone harms you, distance is necessary in order to gain clarity. That's how it works.

---

[6]

WHAT IS HOPE-IUM?

"WHAT THE HECK is hope-ium?" I mentioned it earlier but let me explain. Let's say Sharon is a heroin addict. She's mainlining [8] and shooting up because she is 100 percent controlled by her addiction. This behavior has devastating effects on her life and the people who love her. Sharon lies to herself and to the people around her to protect herself from the truth of what her life has become. "Hope-ium" is a drug that women in emotionally abusive relationships use to avoid facing the truth. Hope-ium is a form of false self-protection used subconsciously to kill the pain of the harm that is being done to you.

How does someone take hope-ium? If you're in an abusive relationship with your husband, spouse, parents, or anyone else, instead of living in the truth of the situation, you are shooting up hope-ium.

Hope-ium is what makes you think, *Well, he really didn't mean it. Maybe I'm being too sensitive*, giving him the benefit of the doubt. Hope-ium is believing what you hope the relationship to be rather than what it actually is. Each time you think these things, you mainline more hope-ium. The more hope-ium you take, the sicker you become. Hope-ium keeps you in denial and makes it impossible for you to see reality.

You're using hope-ium like a drug. It keeps you going and gets you to the next day. Just like any drug, in order to get off of hope-ium, you're going to have to go through withdrawal.

---

*In order to get off of hope-ium,
you're going to have to go through withdrawal.*

You must start living in the truth and withdraw from the thing that you've been doing to mainline hope-ium. Withdrawal is not easy. In fact, it's going to get very difficult because you're going to start seeing your abuser for who they are. You are no longer going to want to take a shot of hope-ium by giving them the benefit of the doubt or making excuses for them. Instead, you're going to see their behavior for what it is and say, "That was extremely hurtful."

What does it look like to detox from hope-ium? You may start to fear the future and the potential harm that may come to you and/or your children. You may feel exhausted,

[6] WHAT IS HOPE-IUM?

overwhelmed, and sad, unsure of who you are as a person. You are also unsure whose version of reality you can trust, so you may bounce between trusting your gut and believing the lies of the person harming you. Waves of grief will hit on what you thought was but no longer is. You may wonder if there really is a God and where He has been during all the chaos and harm, or, you over-spiritualize in an effort to avoid the pain.

Every person's withdrawal will look different. Above are just a few examples. Pay attention to what is happening to you and remember to document. Detoxing from hope-ium is painful. But detoxing from hope-ium is also important. When your system is free of the drug, you will be able to accept the truth and function more efficiently in your life.

During my years working in drug rehab, when someone came in off the street with a long-term heroin addiction, we made them go through detox. For the next three to five days, their life was abjectly miserable. They were in intense physical pain. All they wanted to do was get away from us and go get some more heroin. They struggled and struggled. The last place they wanted to be was in detox.

However, on the other side of those detox days, they transformed into a different person. Suddenly, their reason returned. Their body calmed down. They had a measure of peace and could finally sleep. Their mental clarity returned. They were in a difficult spot but finally had real hope because they were no longer controlled by something outside of them.

It's a very similar situation for those of us who have been in abusive relationships. There is a period of detox that's required, and you *have* to stop taking hope-ium in order to begin the detox process. Hope-ium only keeps you from seeing reality and living in the truth.

Dealers

Every heroin addict has dealers, so do hope-ium addicts. You have to identify your hope-ium dealers. Yes, you have hope-ium dealers! But your hope-ium dealers are notoriously well-intentioned and misinformed.

The key distinction of a hope-ium dealer is that they *don't* believe you are being harmed or abused. They say things like, "Just forgive him" or "God hates divorce no matter what is happening in the marriage." They may give you reading material to better your marriage and encourage you to reconcile like "the others" do. Rather than listening to the harm you are experiencing, they have an agenda to keep your marriage together. No matter who the person is or what position they hold in your life—your pastor, your mom, your best friend—do not allow them to harm you with more hope-ium.

Acceptance

Something I see all the time with women in harmful, toxic, abusive relationships is deep denial about how bad their situation really is. They keep justifying their situation to bolster their hope. But in reality, what they're doing is living in denial.

[6] WHAT IS HOPE-IUM?

If this describes you, then you, too, are living on hope-ium. If you want to be free, you cannot live in denial. Denial kills freedom. Denial kills any kind of honest relationship. You think denial is giving you hope, but it's actually killing real hope by keeping everything buried.

How can you stop dosing yourself with hope-ium? By living in the reality of the situation you were actually in, not the one you hope for. This is why I encourage documentation—the more you externalize (put on paper, talk to someone who you can trust) your actual situation, the clearer you'll become thus living more in reality and less in denial.

Sometimes the people you're surrounded by are the reason it's difficult to accept the reality of your situation. You may have work friends, church friends, or even family members telling you it's your job to make the relationship work. You may hear things like:

- "I know what you need to do. I know how to fix your relationship problem."
- "It can't be that bad. He seems like such a nice guy. Everybody likes him."
- "You know, the Lord hates divorce, and divorce destroys children."
- "Here's what you're going to do. Cook him better meals, be kinder, and have more sex."
- "If you were more patient, everything would be fine."

- "What's the worst thing that can happen? He kills you and you can go be with Jesus." (This statement was the most unbelievable one and was said to a woman by her pastor! Keep in mind her husband put her in the hospital twice.)

These people, your hope-ium dealers, mean well. They want you to be happy and honestly think they know what's going on. They believe that if you take their advice, everything will work out. Well, it's all *really bad advice* and full of the ingredients that are keeping you hooked on hope-ium. The above advice keeps you from looking at the reality of the harm that's being done to you. You use spiritual terms to gloss over the abuse, thus continuing the harm that's happening to you and your children.

Living in the Truth

Living in the truth means experiencing pain and grief. Pain is a reality of living in the truth. That's why we avoid it. It's like sticking your hand in a buzz saw.

Who wants to do that?

No one!

How do you know if you're *not* living in the truth? The evidence might sound something like, "Well, I just wanted to give him the benefit of the doubt." My response is, "Okay, for what, the four-hundredth time? How many times are you going to give him 'the benefit of the doubt?' Is there a rule?"

[6] WHAT IS HOPE-IUM?

Unfortunately, within many churches, the oft-unspoken but understood rule for women is, "You will *indefinitely* give him the benefit of the doubt." That is *not* a healthy way to live.

I've said it before, and I'll say it again: Document the behavior you see on a regular basis. This is going to help you get off hope-ium, start living in the truth, and guide you toward acceptance of your situation. It's also going to reveal how much hope-ium you're taking. Hope-ium will *not* lead you to a resolution in your relationship.

Remember your gut? Think back and be honest if you've been in a situation like this: Your husband is talking to you, but your gut says, *Oh … this is not right. This is not what I want. No!*

Have you ever become fearful? Your palms were sweating, and you were filled with fear of what he might do? Is that something you should document? Is that something real, or is it something you're going to gloss over and deny?

Hope-ium. Denial. Glossing over. These are all justifications that are building up the abusive dynamic in your relationship. If you don't start living in the truth, you're going to continue to give power to your abuser.

> *If you don't start living in the truth, you're going to continue to give power to your abuser.*

However, if you start living in the truth instead of denial, you are going to experience pain. It's a hard truth but remember that pain is your number-one goal. You must understand that you're going to have to move into the pain. Acceptance of the pain and *not* taking hope-ium will lead you to freedom.

You must understand that you're going to have to move into the pain. Acceptance of the pain and not taking hope-ium will lead you to freedom.

Well-meaning people at church will tell you that it's your job to make your abuser "less bad." They will give your abuser the benefit of the doubt and spiritualize your situation. That is *not* from God. If you're going to be in a healthy relationship, you cannot think that way.

Be honest with yourself as you document. It will feel uncomfortable. The reality of the abusive relationship is very unhealthy. As you start to recognize reality, you will feel pain, but the pain is a good thing. You *will* get to the other side of the pain. But acceptance and living in the truth of your situation are the first goals. Every abusive relationship is unique, so stepping into the pain looks different for everyone.

Something else that is common among women living in abusive relationships is comparison: "Oh, my situation isn't as bad as hers." But pain looks different for everyone, so comparison only leads to a very bad place. No one ever wins in the game of comparison. Do you compare your situation with

[6] WHAT IS HOPE-IUM?

others? Stop comparing and start examining and validating your own situation.

Perhaps the best place to start is to watch how your kids are being treated. You might be able to see the abuse more clearly in them in order to apply it to yourself. Wherever you start, you must look at your situation honestly instead of denying, rationalizing, minimizing, justifying, spiritualizing, and avoiding. These are all tactics that keep you stuck in the abusive relationship. The way out is through looking at reality as it is, not as you wish it to be. Once you start to see your situation clearly, find someone to talk with whom you can trust. This healthy relationship will help you live in the truth of your situation, which involves accepting the pain. Pain is step one in getting to the door of freedom. As you face the pain, you become strong and less manipulatable.

> *As you face the pain,*
> *you become strong*
> *and less manipulatable.*

In *The Road Less Traveled*, M. Scott Peck wrote, "The attempt to avoid legitimate suffering lies at the root of all emotional illness … What makes life difficult is that the process of confronting and solving problems is a difficult one. Yet it is only because of problems that we grow mentally and spiritually."[9] As we discussed earlier, avoidance gives power to the abuser. If you want to take power from the abuser, you have to get to the truth of your situation. You *can* get to the other side. I'm living proof you can do it. I've also talked to thousands of other women who have gotten to the other side.

"Be strong and courageous," as they say in church, but take it one day at a time. You're not going to eat this elephant all at once. Today, just today, document one thing. Get one piece of clarity—that's all. All through this healing process, try to remember *change is a process, not an event*. You're not going to change all at once. You're going to do one thing today. One documentation. You don't have to save the world. You're not going to change your relationship all at once. Just do one thing today. Remember that tomorrow is another chance to do one more thing.

Change is a process, not an event.
You're not going to change all at once.

How to Live in the Truth

I've introduced you to the concept of hope-ium, which is what we use to avoid the truth of our situation. I've also touched on living in the truth, but what exactly does that look like? How does living in the truth change your reality? When you're in a destructive or abusive relationship, one of the first things you have to be willing to do is let the relationship die.

[6] WHAT IS HOPE-IUM?

If you're trying to make the abusive relationship work, it will be easier for your abuser to manipulate you. This is because you're putting lots of energy into an outcome you have no control over. In any relationship, you only have control over one side, but in an abusive relationship, you have an abuser telling you the relational problems are your fault. "If you would just do A, then B would happen. If you would just do A, then I wouldn't have to do C." Everything becomes your fault.

You're putting all your energy into forcing this abusive relationship to work, but it never will. It's a waste of energy. You have to be willing to let go of the relationship, get a divorce, separate, and stop communicating with your abuser. You must be willing to deal with the reality of their harm by letting the relationship go.

GIVING CPR TO A DEAD GUY

I have seen it in movies. A loved one dies, and a family member starts giving them CPR. Many times, they keep giving CPR even though the person is clearly dead. They just keep pumping until someone says, "Hey, man, it's okay. Let it go. Stop. They're gone."

The family member is giving CPR not to help the person (because they are clearly dead) but because they don't want to face the pain and grief of losing their loved one. The CPR they're doing is actually about them, not the dead person. I see this all the time in abusive relationships. The person who is being abused keeps giving CPR to the dead guy. When a

DEATH OF A THOUSAND CUTS

woman comes to me looking for help, usually the relationship has been "dead" for a long time, and she is hoping I can breathe life back into it. She is asking *me* to give CPR to the dead guy!

You must assess the death of the relationship and begin to live in the truth of that death—no excuses. I say that because women have given me numerous excuses:

"Well, you know, I can't get a divorce. I'm a Christian."

"I can't get a divorce. I don't have any money."

"I can't get a divorce because of the kids."

"I can't confront him. He'll harm me. He'll take my money and make me miserable."

All of these things can happen. I'm not saying these reasons aren't valid or terrifying. But it's important to live in the truth of what your relationship is and see that you do have choices. Assess the death of your relationship, and live in the truth of that death.

*Assess the death of your relationship,
and live in the truth of that death.*

[6] WHAT IS HOPE-IUM?

Here are some signs that you're in a dead marriage:

- You realize that you're the only one making an effort to improve the marriage.
- It feels like you're on a bicycle built for two with only one person pedaling.
- You fantasize about your partner dying and you being free.
- When you're depressed, you imagine running away from it all.
- You find yourself emotionally or physically connecting with another member of the opposite sex on a deep level.
- You don't want to go home because he is there.
- There is no talk or action regarding "us," only him.
- The idea of having sex with him makes you sick to your stomach.
- He stops dating you and is never romantic.
- You are the one planning most of the experiences together to keep the relationship alive.
- You don't see behavior from him that says, "I love you" and "I see you."
- The words "I love you" are on autopilot with no meaning attached.

DEATH OF A THOUSAND CUTS

- Your anniversary is just a number on the calendar, nothing to celebrate.

- Regardless of how clear you are that his behavior is hurting you, he doesn't stop or have empathy for the pain he is causing.

- You notice that he would rather watch pornography than have sex with you.

To find freedom, you must be willing to consider the death of your relationship both emotionally and spiritually. Ask yourself these questions about your relationship:

- Do I feel emotionally safe?

- Am I afraid of him?

- Do I have physical intimacy? If I do, then is it harmful, painful, or one-sided?

- Do I have emotional intimacy?

- Am I afraid to talk to him?

- Does he take responsibility?

- Is he emotionally trustworthy?

If you can look your relationship in the face and see that it's dead, unhealthy, or in the process of dying, then you will be freed to start the work of healing. Instead of wasting energy

[6] WHAT IS HOPE-IUM?

giving CPR to a dead guy, you'll be able to spend your energy accepting the truth.

If you're reading this book, then it is likely you have already suffered a great deal of harm. Your relationship may already be dead. I can't give you advice on how to give CPR to a dead guy. But I can give you advice on how to make sure that you're well and that you're living in a healthy state.

NOT YOUR RESPONSIBILITY

In an abusive relationship, you are repeatedly told that you're the problem. One of the first things you must do is stop taking responsibility for what is not yours. Remember the idea that you can only be responsible for yourself? You cannot be responsible for someone else's behavior. If your spouse is telling you it's your fault for how they behave, please realize they are lying. You can *never* be responsible for someone else's behavior.

> *Stop taking responsibility*
> *for what is not yours.*

I've talked about the importance of documenting your abuser's actions since Chapter 2, and I will continue to talk about it because it's *critical*. Something I haven't mentioned is that you can show your documentation to a third party. It's almost impossible to accurately recall the significant conversations with your abuser because you can't possibly remember all that was said.

It doesn't matter how you do it, just keep documenting. This practice will reveal the actual nature of the relationship—what it really is. As you start to accept that truth, you're going to gain more clarity, and as the clarity comes, you'll need to make difficult decisions about what to do next.

Once you accept the truth that your relationship is unhealthy, you're likely going to experience some fear, anger, and uncertainty. These emotions are the reason why you have avoided the truth and shot hope-ium into your veins. Avoiding reality does not provide room for hope. The hope of healing comes from accepting the truth.

> *The hope of healing comes from accepting the truth.*

I wish the truth wasn't hard to accept. I wish the truth *wasn't* that you have an abusive relationship. I *wish* the truth was that your spouse was not abusive. But wishing doesn't change anything. Accepting the truth and living within it is how we start to navigate to heal. You cannot find healing with avoidance.

For example, if I go to the hospital and have open heart surgery, what would people expect of me once I returned home? Would they expect me to function like I did before the day I went in? No. They would expect me to have a period of

[6] WHAT IS HOPE-IUM?

recovery. Why should it be any different for emotional heart surgery? That's what beginning to accept the truth is like: emotional heart surgery. A recovery period is to be expected. You're going to be physically tired, feel overwhelmed, and experience uncomfortable emotions. It will feel like it's all too much, and you may even want to go back to the way things were. It will feel that way because the truth of your relationship is becoming clear.

When you address an abusive relationship, you're supposed to feel uncomfortable. You must be willing to sacrifice what's most precious to you or it will control you. If this describes you, you're in the right place. It's *not* comfortable, nor should it be. If you're feeling comfortable, it's because you're still in denial. When you address an abusive relationship, it's natural for you to feel uncomfortable.

Many women in abusive relationships are fearful of letting go of that relationship because they believe letting go is wrong. But how can it be wrong to get rid of something that's destroying you? Even if no one else can see it, the *fact* is that you are being destroyed. Remember, emotional abuse leads to the destruction of your soul.

Emotional abuse leads to the destruction of your soul.

DEATH OF A THOUSAND CUTS

[7]

GRIEF & DOCUMENTATION

IF YOU'RE IN an abusive relationship, you likely experience or carry a lot of grief inside. This section will focus specifically on the grief that comes from being in an abusive relationship. One of the first things that starts to happen as you grieve is that you realize your grief is about *what you're not getting* and what you don't have. The grief you feel is for all the dreams you had for the relationship. No one stands at the altar and says, "Here's to being miserable and tortured." When you understand what is happening to you—such as being harmed, living in an unhealthy or even dangerous relationship—it brings up a lot of grief.

Grieving the death of the relationship, and the specific issues that existed within that relationship, will come *after* you get clear about what has been happening. However, when people start to examine their grief, their first reaction is to jump right back into their coping mechanisms:

- Avoid
- Rationalize
- Minimize
- Justify
- Deny
- Spiritualize

If you tend to choose one of these coping mechanisms, you will spend energy on something that's going to lead you to *stay* in the relationship. This will only prolong the grieving process. One of the ways to get out of the relationship is to grieve sooner. I understand that grieving is an undesirable state. We all want to avoid it. Grief doesn't make sense. But grieving the death of your relationship sooner rather than later will help you find freedom more quickly.

The kind of grief I'm talking about is *not* like the grief of a loved one who dies. It's more like a death without a funeral. The person is still alive, but the relationship is dead. Furthermore, they are still with you on a daily basis, or at least interacting with you on a regular basis, and the relationship is causing you harm.

[7] GRIEF & DOCUMENTATION

Start looking at the death of your relationship and acknowledge it internally. Let those feelings of grief surface. Let the loss sink in. Your grief of the loss of the relationship is essential to your freedom. And the freedom you seek is on the other side of the grief.

> *Your grief of the loss of the relationship is essential to your freedom. And the freedom you seek is on the other side of the grief.*

M. Scott Peck's teachings helped me understand that the avoidance of pain is the beginning of all unhealthy behavior. In order to change our life and heal, we must venture into this uneasy terrain. We all try to avoid pain, but I'm going to challenge you here. Think about what is causing you to feel discomfort. Where is the pain coming from? Embrace it. Don't avoid it. If you embrace the pain one out of the ten times you are given the opportunity, then great. You're not going to be able do it every time because you've been "trained" not to do so in your abusive relationship. Your spouse has trained you to avoid the pain. If you don't see it, you won't feel it. So let that ugly stuff come to the surface as it's crucial for your healing.

Here's an example of what it might look like to embrace the pain. During your day, a memory surfaces of a conversation you had the day before with your abuser. Maybe you tried to resolve something, and the other person dodged it. Maybe they just badgered you, keeping you up all night talking to you about it to convince you *not* to think the way you think. Some time passes. But the next day, you're doing the dishes, or driving your car, or lying in bed, and the memory surfaces. What do you do at that moment? Do you begin the mental gymnastics of pushing it down? Or do you embrace it and start documenting?

Yes, there's that word again, *document*. Start documenting those moments of grief and then *feel* the grief. Begin by letting those feelings in and accepting them. The next step is you must *express* the emotions that go with the grief. *Tears are the blood of the soul.* If you cut your arm, what's the first thing that happens? You bleed. That makes bleeding the first stage of healing. If your soul is cut, what is the first stage of healing? Letting your tears out. Allow your emotions to surface. In doing so, you validate your wound by expressing the appropriate corresponding emotions. Be willing to move into the pain.

Tears are the blood of the soul.

A lot of women waste precious energy on avoidance. But imagine putting that energy into the grief and letting it out. It feels counterintuitive. It feels right to avoid grief so you can save your strength. But letting the grief out is going to give you *more* strength on the other side than avoiding it will.

For many people, the family's pathology, or the system they are living in with their spouse, doesn't allow them to express those emotions. Everything must be suppressed. Suppression,

[7] GRIEF & DOCUMENTATION

suppression, suppression! If one little tear is let out, then you're breaking the rules of the system.

- Grief *is* breaking the system and is a healthy response.
- Grieving is good for your relationship with your spouse and your children.

When you grieve, what you're doing is giving value to yourself. By seeing the pain, you are saying, "What has happened to me is important." Grieving allows you to prioritize your self-worth and your value.

Grief, sadness, regret, and loss are going to emerge, so expect those emotions. They will help you recognize what you're dealing with. *Let it out!* As you go through the process of grieving, you'll eventually move into healing. Remember, grieving is just the beginning. You're not going to stay there or be trapped there. I promise you won't die in grief, but emotionally speaking, you will die if you avoid it.

Document Your Grief

I am often asked, "Why should I document my grief? It seems like an exercise in hurting myself." Good question! I believe that documenting the details of what's going on in the grief process is imperative to your healing. You are living in a relationship where nothing is as it seems. There has been a lot of rationalizing, minimizing, and justifying your partner's abusive behavior. You're in a smoke-and-mirrors situation where you cannot see or live in the truth. So instead, you spend your days trying to manage the abuse and the lies.

Being in an abusive relationship causes you to suppress what your gut is saying. Your gut is what's going to lead you out of this, not your head.

Being in an abusive relationship causes you to suppress what your gut is saying. Your gut is what's going to lead you out of this, not your head.

Pulling away, getting to a quiet place, and documenting your grief will give you space to *feel* what's going on. It is crucial to listen to your gut instead of your head. Your head is full of the lies you've been fed over many years by the toxic person you're living with. Documenting the grief will help you sort out the lies and see the truth clearly.

When you sit down and become quiet, painful feelings begin to emerge. Feeling overwhelmed and uncomfortable, your first instinct is to shut down. This is how you survived being in an abusive relationship.

Getting some time away to let yourself feel the pain and grief may be difficult. You probably won't want to do it. No one sits down and says, "Oh, I can't wait to document the pain going on inside of me." That's not how humans work.

[7] GRIEF & DOCUMENTATION

As difficult as documenting may be, let that stuff come up and write it down. Write whatever comes up—and *no editing!* It takes time, and it may feel risky, but it is worth the time and risk. When you are documenting grief, your job is *not* to figure it out. Your job is *not* to understand it. Your job is just to document it.

As we discussed previously, make sure that when you document, you have a way to keep it private and to *keep you safe*. You do not want anything you document to be discovered. I've experimented with this for myself. For me, sometimes writing is best. Sometimes typing works, whether I use my Notes app (with a password) on my phone, or if I click away on my computer and place the document in a password-protected file. Sometimes I like using voice memos. It doesn't matter what you use, just do *something*, and make sure no one can access it.

When I write with a pen or pencil, physically putting the words on paper, I feel it's a very different emotional process than typing. There is something about documenting in my own handwriting that feels very safe and generates authenticity in my writing. Most of the time, no one can read what I've written, including me. It's like trying to read hieroglyphics. Even I have to decode it when I go back to read it a month or so later.

Focus on whatever form of documentation enables you to express your honest feelings. Your abuser's training tells you *not* to be honest. So take the opportunity to document as often as you can. I know you don't want to do this. Sometimes you are going to have opportunities to document that you fail to take.

You're going to feel resistant. Just accept these moments, and don't view failure and resistance as problems. See them as a natural part of the healing process.

THE COMMITTEE IN YOUR MIND

You will sometimes have a feeling or feelings come up out of nowhere. It's unconscious, it just happens. For example, you feel remorse. You don't like to feel remorse, so you push it away. I call the voices in your head "the committee." Just as in life, every committee in your mind has a chairman. You need to discover who the chairman of your committee is. In my case, it is my dad. When the committee in my head gets going, I still hear my dad saying, "You're not good enough!" or "You're stupid!" The chairman of your committee is probably your abuser. His voice has trained you to think this way and to doubt your own experiences. But the truth is, your abuser has harmed you. *He* is the problem, not you.

The committee in your mind will eventually bring the feelings of abuse back to you, only now they are not the same feelings as when you experienced them the first time. Now, they are connected to other things. The remorse comes back, coupled with shame. The emotions are compounding. So you push those feelings away again. But it's not over... The committee brings them back up. And again, there's something new attached. Now the remorse brings with it both shame and fear. This might happen five, ten, or one hundred times. How are you ever going to have any clarity or peace? It's like the

[7] GRIEF & DOCUMENTATION

committee has put your feelings on an emotional Lazy Susan, bringing them around again and again, waving their fingers at you each time the emotions surface.

The way to stop the committee is to document what you feel the first time you feel it. In two weeks, when you look back at that feeling you documented, it will be exactly the same. It hasn't changed or compounded. The committee has not been able to add anything to it, and you will be able to recognize the lies of the chairman of the committee.

This practice of documenting will give you context for your feelings. In an abusive relationship, documenting helps you gain perspective on what is actually happening by freeing you from compounding emotions.

> *The practice of documenting gives you context for your feelings. In an abusive relationship, documenting helps you gain perspective on what is actually happening.*

Documenting will also lead you to a place of healing, but you can't get there without the documentation of those thoughts and feelings. You're not going to wake up one morning and be motivated and ready to document your pain and grief. You're going to want to avoid it. But remember, avoidance will harm you and elongate the process of your healing.

DEATH OF A THOUSAND CUTS

What Should I Document?

You might also document:

- Losses you feel.
- That you feel unloved or are afraid of your spouse.
- The harm your children are experiencing.
- The difficult relationships you have with your in-laws or the people at church.
- The fear you feel when you're afraid to say anything about what's actually happening in your life.

When those experiences or feelings rise to the surface, begin at that place. If you're in an emotionally abusive relationship, you *have* losses. That's the place for you to start.

Do you feel sad, lost, afraid, angry, hurt, overwhelmed, or tired? Those are the feelings to document. Even if you're feeling the same thing all the time, just keep writing it down. Even if it feels redundant, keep doing it because if you feel the same way all the time, that means there's probably some consistent unhealthiness in your life. Documenting regularly will reveal consistent behavioral patterns in your relationship with an abusive person. And often, there are indeed consistent behavioral patterns in an abusive relationship.

[7] GRIEF & DOCUMENTATION

Often, there are consistent behavioral patterns in an abusive relationship.

A question I hear often is, "How long should I wait to review what I have written?" Well, there is no right answer to that. When you review your documentation, don't try to fix it or change anything. Just let it be. Let the consequences of your reality come to the surface.

For example, if you see a pattern of documenting how afraid you are of your spouse, don't look at that record and start making plans on how to not be afraid. Instead, say, "Wow, I'm afraid of my spouse. That's horrible. That's not what I came into this relationship for. That's not what I want. That really causes me pain."

Be with the reality you have documented. Don't try to fix it, avoid it, sugarcoat it, spiritualize it, deny it, rationalize it, or minimize it. Being with your reality is going to be the way you come out of the situation. By being with it, you're accepting the truth. And *the truth* is what's going to move you into freedom, not avoidance.

The truth is what's going to move you into freedom, not avoidance.

WHY IS GRIEF IMPORTANT?

Grief is important because without it, you'll stay stuck in a harmful, toxic, and unhealthy situation. Grief is a mercy because it's helping you to accept and identify a problem. Let's say you identify that your spouse is emotionally abusive. If that doesn't produce grief, then you're still in denial. You want to move out of denial because when you stay there, it's like taking hope-ium. And without grief, the result is more pressure, pain, and loss (loss of your future). Grief is a profoundly important process to free you from what's happening. I know it's very difficult, but it's even more valuable than hope at first.

RIDING THE WAVES OF GRIEF

Grief is not something you can control. It comes in waves. Recall my personal story. There were days after my marriage ended when I felt somewhat normal, and other days where I was doubled over in the fetal position because of grief. I could never predict what would make one day worse than the next. The key to surviving the waves of grief was to let myself feel each bump. There is no timeframe anyone can give you. The time it takes to grieve will be specific to your context.

> *Grief is not something you can control.*
> *It comes in waves.*

[7] GRIEF & DOCUMENTATION

One minute, you might be fine. The next minute, you're in bed, immobile. That's how grief works. You can't control how or when it comes, but when it does, let yourself feel it. Even if you can only let yourself feel the grief one out of ten times, let it come. That's a start. It means you are making progress.

One of the consequences of avoiding grief is that internal pressure builds up. Nothing ever gets resolved. Anxiety, depression, helplessness, and intense physical pain can occur because of the built-up pressure. The body, mind, and spirit can't deal with the unresolved grief. We're not designed to avoid resolution.

Another consequence of holding on to emotional pain is having less energy and a shorter fuse. Think of it this way: Your internal emotional space should be the size of a gallon of milk. But because you're living in denial and the grief is so high, the emotional space you have available is the size of just a *drop* of milk. Your emotional space is too limited. You can't function. You can't hold all of the emotional content you are experiencing.

This lack of emotional space is felt even more intensely if your kids are having a bad day, if someone else behaves badly, or if someone cuts you off in traffic. You just have no emotional space to handle things like this. And it's not because you did something wrong, it's because you're being harmed. And when you start to grieve, you're *giving* yourself emotional space even though it feels like the opposite, like the energy you're using to grieve, the energy used to feel the emotions, is *taking* space, not *giving* space. To the contrary, when you start to grieve, you're *giving* yourself emotional space.

Grief is physically draining. I went through severe grief after being separated once I recognized how bad the reality of my situation was. I was physically exhausted because that kind of emotional expression drains you. Eventually, you'll notice little things, like the tightness in your chest has relaxed a little and you can breathe. Allowing yourself to express the grief has given you space because you're honoring the reality of your pain.

The feeling of exhaustion may take time to subside before you feel your emotional space increase. But don't confuse the feeling of exhaustion with depression as you wait. The exhaustion is a natural consequence. When you grieve, you're going to feel physically drained. You have been living in a situation where you have been pressured to "be okay." You've been trained to take care of everything and make it all happen. You have been programmed to "not have a bad day."

THINGS YOU MIGHT BE GRIEVING

One of the things you will grieve is the loss of relationships—with your kids, their dad, your family, your in-laws, and yourself. You're going to grieve the loss of the dream you had when you stood at the altar and thought, *This is going to be magnificent! He's so wonderful! This is everything I've ever dreamed of!* At least that's what I hope you were thinking on your wedding day. Most of us don't get married because we're looking to be

[7] GRIEF & DOCUMENTATION

harmed. But years later, all of the effort and hard work hasn't changed anything. I hear it all the time: "I gave *so* much effort over *so* many years. I poured myself into this relationship."

But let's get *real* right now: If the relationship could have been fixed by your effort, it would have been fixed by now. No amount of effort is going to fix the relationship. The issue doesn't lie with you. This understanding ushers in a lot of grief over time lost, life wasted, and lost hope.

> *No amount of effort is going to fix the relationship. The issue doesn't lie with you. This understanding ushers in a lot of grief over time lost, life wasted, and lost hope.*

Separation is a huge loss, and that is before considering the kids and what may happen to them. You might say, "Oh no! Are they going to be like him?" To some degree, yes, they will. They can't avoid it. As you go through this process, my hope is that you'll have other people around you who understand what you've been going through. People like this really help the healing process run more smoothly. If you're all alone and isolated, separation is going to be a much more difficult task. Success is possible, but you'll have to tackle a higher hurdle.

Surround yourself with people who understand what you're going through and who can validate what you are saying, or at least listen without denying your reality. Find people who will validate that you are not crazy. Remember, the person you're living with has told you over and over that everything bad that happens is your fault: "You're the problem. You're crazy and overly sensitive." The overall message is that you are not enough. As you go through the healing process, the lies from your abuser are going to surface and trigger you. Remember the wagging finger of the committee in your head. Doing so will remind you that those voices are false.

When you can talk with someone who understands, they will validate what you're going through. If they truly understand, they have probably been in a similar situation to yours. They can share what happened to them and give you hope that they're okay and didn't die. Just hearing and knowing someone had success in leaving their abuser and starting a new life is so helpful. It's good to have a safe place where you can talk about your situation.

How Can I Tell if I am Avoiding Grief?

Remember when we discussed emotional internal pressure? That's how you know you're avoiding grief. You have *a lot* of internal pressure but not a lot of internal peace. There's very little space for anything to happen emotionally (the drop of milk). You're down, overwhelmed, tense, always waiting for the other shoe to fall. You feel exhausted and sometimes you don't want to go on. Many times, you're looking for a way to escape by doing harmful behaviors: overeating, over-drinking, isolating yourself, overworking, dodging emotions, smoking, doing drugs, or taking medication you don't need. When you

[7] GRIEF & DOCUMENTATION

have a very strong desire to check out, this is a signal you're avoiding grief.

WHO IS THE PERSON RESPONSIBLE FOR DEFINING THE GRIEF?

You and no one else define what you grieve. In American culture, and particularly in Christian culture, it's a different story. We're told what we're *allowed* to grieve for and what we're *not*. For instance, you're hurting about the death of your dream—your family and your marriage is being destroyed. But when you talk with someone at church, they say, "Don't worry. Don't fret." But the truth is, you decide what to grieve because you're *valuable*. When you have the power to decide, you value yourself enough to *not* avoid pain. Instead, you can let yourself hurt and say, "This situation is not okay with me!"

Remember these two rules:

1) No crazy allowed!
2) You get to determine what is crazy. You also get to decide what is causing you grief and harm.

It doesn't matter what the pastor says, what your husband says, or what your mother, brother, in-laws, sister, or kids say. What *you say* is what matters. This is a vital part of you starting to live a healthy life. You must be honest about what's happening to you, allowing that realization come, and then validating it by being in it.

You are worth it!

The pain that you're experiencing is a sign that you're starting to value yourself instead of denying, deflecting, and rationalizing.

Will My Life Fall Apart if I Start to Grieve?

If you start to grieve, you might feel like you are never going to come back. For example, you might be thinking, *If I go into that rabbit hole of grief, I might never get out. There's just too much there. I'll be overwhelmed, incapacitated, and unable to get through it.*

I understand completely. Let me give you an analogy that might help you. Years ago, one of my good friends had a twenty-two-year-old son who had recently graduated from college. Tragically, he died in an accident at a national park. He was on his way to getting his PhD so he could help people. He wanted to be a counselor. His dad and mom are beautiful people with a great family. There was unbelievable grief at the tragic death of their son. It was beyond difficult for them.

I was talking to his mom after the tragedy, and she was still deep in grief. One of the things I said to her was, "You know, you really have to work at accepting this."

She said, "I am never going to accept that my son died! What I have to do is live with it the best I can."

[7] GRIEF & DOCUMENTATION

I had to admit her reasoning. Who wants to accept that their child died tragically? She was never going to forget what happened.

So what *does* it mean to grieve something like the death of a child? One of the things she shared was truly amazing. She said at first the grief was a pit she had fallen into and felt she would never get out of. "It's just too much. My son is dead. I can't handle this. It's overwhelming. I can't even look at it. I can't do it."

"I understand," was my simple response.

She continued, "Over time, I realized that grief is not a pit, it's a tunnel. You enter the tunnel and all you can see is darkness. You can't see the other side. You have no idea what's in that tunnel. You have no idea how you're going to get to the other side. You have no idea what's going to happen to you *in* that tunnel."

You need to have some other people with you in the tunnel. Their presence is very important because they're going to help you get to the other side. *On the other side of the grief is the freedom you seek.* You're going to enter the tunnel, but you're not going to die there. You're not going to get stuck there. You're going to walk through it. Once you are on the other side, you're going to have freedom.

One of the most powerful things you can do when you've been abused is to *face the pain of what happened to you and then walk through it.* If you don't grieve, your avoidance and denial give your abuser power. But on the other side of the tunnel, you will not be able to be manipulated.

[8]

DETOX

EARLIER, I BRIEFLY spoke about a period of required detox. In the process of becoming aware you're with someone who's toxic, you need to detox from the relationship that's causing you harm. In this chapter, I'm going to give you a clearer image of what detox looks like.

In the context of emotional and spiritual abuse, *detox* is a process of painful withdrawal. But on the other side is clarity and the opportunity to live your life dramatically differently. You're unhappy, overwhelmed, sad, broken, hopeless, hurt—and it doesn't seem to stop. There's no way to get away from it. Everything you try fails. You can't get the abuser to acknowledge anything. You can't get them to take responsibility for anything. They're relentless, unkind, and self-centered as they rationalize, minimize, justify, deny, and spiritualize their abusive behavior. And you want ... *out*.

Detox is one of the first things that has to happen, and detox is always going to happen because of some kind of boundary. I will go into detail in this and the next chapter on what setting a boundary looks like. Remember that a hope-ium addict is like a heroin addict. When a heroin addict comes to detox for four or five days, their life feels miserable. They want to stop doing detox and go get some heroin to end the pain.

To get healthy, you have to go through the process of detox so that on the other side you actually have a choice about how you want to live. In a toxic relationship, it becomes *your job* to make it work. Your state of mind becomes, "How do I keep this going? How do I protect the kids? How do I make him not get upset? If I was only happier, less of a nag, prettier, spontaneous, or I wasn't so sad and sensitive, then he would get better."

No. Your situation is unlikely to change—not in an emotionally abusive relationship.

The problem is the person you're in the relationship with has what I call "malignant denial." Malignant means this denial is going to produce death. Their denial is so intact, it's going to create emotional death. That's what you're experiencing. For you to get better, you can't continue the mental gymnastics or come at it from another angle. You have to get away from it. Detox will require, at a minimum, less communication with the person who is toxic.

[8] DETOX

> *Detox will require, at a minimum, less communication with the person who is toxic.*

How do you accomplish that? Many women have said to me, "I'm married to the person. How am I supposed to detox from him?" Though it may seem impossible, the good news is that there are many ways to do it. Begin with writing a letter of resignation to yourself, *effective immediately*. Resign from managing your abuser and trying to make him well. It's impossible for you to do that anyway.

If anybody could "make" them well by sheer effort, you probably would have done so by now. You've poured out excessive amounts of effort and tried to make it work. You have bent yourself into unhealthy shapes and forms for your abuser. But no matter how hard you try, or how you try to shape yourself around the other person, your efforts are not going to change anything. *Your efforts don't matter.* When you're in a relationship with someone who has so much malignant denial, that person believes their own lies.

> *When you're in a relationship with someone who has so much malignant denial, that person believes their own lies.*

DEATH OF A THOUSAND CUTS

Your spouse will look you straight in the eye and say something that you *know* is a lie, but they are convinced of their truth and believe their lie so deeply that it leaves you feeling confused. This is a pattern within emotional abuse that you must start detoxing from. If you do not, this toxic pattern is going to keep contaminating you. You're going to keep spinning out and feeling overwhelmed. When the toxic lies are present, you never have the fuel needed, the emotional space needed, or the strength needed to fight. You just put all your energy into surviving. Detoxing is imperative, and it starts with recognizing the need to stop focusing on the other person and create *boundaries*.

If he goes out of town for a weekend, document your feelings. When he's gone, do you feel relief, safety, or like you can breathe again? Those feelings are evidence that you need to detox from the relationship. With these feelings documented, you can navigate a plan to deal with setting appropriate boundaries.

Trust Your Gut

It took me a long time to learn how to trust my gut. For better or worse, I was born a very sensitive soul. That's who I am. *But my childhood experiences taught me to suppress my gut instincts because my father was so dangerous.* As a child, I did not believe my sensitivity was a gift.

Do you feel like your sensitivity is the problem in your situation? Your abuser might say, "You're too sensitive. You

[8] DETOX

shouldn't feel that way. You just need to get over it." But this isn't true.

You may even have people in your life who are teaching you to suppress your gut by ignoring your instincts and giving your abuser what he wants. What these people are teaching you to do, whether they realize it or not, is to be abused.

It's your gut that will *lead you out* of this—not your abuser or other people. The problem with your gut is that it gives you information you can't prove. That's a real challenge because in an abusive relationship, everything has to be proven, right? This can be nauseatingly problematic. Layer on a spiritual environment in which you must have a Bible verse to support all of your actions, and your problems only get deeper.

Learning to trust your gut is going to feel very odd in the beginning. You have a lot of training that has taught you *not* to do that. Think of this learning process in terms of moving percentages—you will trust your gut 5 percent more today, then 5 percent more tomorrow. Or start with a more achievable goal, such as listening to your gut one out of ten times at the start.

Most women I talk to say that they experience their instincts the most when they're with their children. It is natural for parents to have their instincts on high alert when their children may be in danger. Therefore abused women tend to pay attention to their instincts with their children more than at any other time. If this is true for you, start there. You deeply love your kids, and they are a safe relationship. Since your instincts are on high alert with them, pay attention to that and start to recognize cues as they arise.

It's helpful to remember that when you are with your abuser, you are in your head, not your gut. That's not going to change easily. When you feel in your gut that something is wrong, try to *immediately* respond to that instinct. Make sure that you're in a safe situation when you do this. Learning to listen to your gut is going to take time, and if you're in a very difficult or dangerous environment, your defense mechanisms are going to be so high you probably won't "hear" your gut anyway.

> *When you are with your abuser,*
> *you are in your head, not your gut.*

When you're in a safer environment, try paying attention to your gut. As you practice this and have positive experiences, you're going to start to realize, "Oh, wow. This is actually very healthy. This is actually very effective." You'll begin to feel an internal congruency. "Oh! I felt that. I thought this and then I did that." Instead of being afraid of your instincts, you'll begin to see the process of how your instincts lead you to safety.

You're going to have to take a risk. What constitutes a risk in an abusive environment? Everything you *don't want to do*. It's when you finally say no to one of the many things he often expects from you. It's when you contact an attorney and learn more about your rights. It's when you choose to walk away from an argument that is going nowhere. It's anything your gut is whispering to you to do but your mind is telling you not to. You're going to have to take a risk at some point in order to break free. Trust your gut instinct and move from there.

Maybe you begin the process of trusting your gut with a girlfriend, boyfriend, or your child to see what it looks and feels like. Your gut is going to give you the information that's going to lead you out. When it does, it's likely going to be information that's difficult to hear.

I was taught that disagreeing with my abuser was wrong or bad, and I shouldn't feel that way. Giving my feelings of disagreement value was a very big hurdle for me to get over. But I eventually learned something that is so very important: *trusting your gut validates you*. It aligns you with your *actual* value as a human being, who was created by God. Why would the God of the universe give you a spirit if you're not valuable, not worthy, not loved, not cared for?

When you trust your gut, you will start to believe the reality of who you are and stop believing the lies that you're being told. Trusting your gut is one of the ways to stop the negative lies from being a factor in your value. In an abusive relationship, you will be told a fundamental lie: *You're* the problem. Don't believe the lie. You might *have* problems, but you're not *the* problem. You're *not* the causal force. Trusting your gut begins the process of undoing that lie.

DEATH OF A THOUSAND CUTS

When you trust your gut, you start to believe the reality of who you are and stop believing the lies you're being told.

You will need a lot of validation to start trusting your gut because everything in your head and the people around you are telling you not to. Document and take some risks. Remember, if you listen to your gut one out of ten times, you're moving forward. But it won't happen unless you take that first risk. It will probably feel like you're jumping off a cliff.

As you take risks, they will reveal a path that you're going to have to take to get out of the relationship. The information is going to come from your gut. It's not something that's written down somewhere or prescribed by an outside source. You are the source. This is another reason why learning to trust your gut is very important.

It's a crucial skill that you *have* to develop. And trusting your gut is an abuser's kryptonite.

Trusting your gut is an abuser's kryptonite.

[9]

HOW TO SET BOUNDARIES YOU CAN KEEP

LIVING IN AN emotionally abusive relationship, boundaries are something you desperately need but are probably afraid of implementing or even asking for. You need them to maintain your emotional health, but you're afraid of them because of the consequences of upsetting your abuser.

Many people I've talked to have this issue: They are generally aware there is a problem. But denial, rationalizing, and minimizing their spouse's toxic behavior causes them to get confused about the boundary structure.

Instead of taking action and drawing a clear boundary regarding what is acceptable and what is unacceptable, many people keep making excuses and give their abuser the benefit of the doubt. Consequently, their will to live gets sucked out a little at a time. This is how to die the death of a thousand cuts: the unwillingness, for many reasons, to establish clear boundary lines.

What a Boundary Looks Like & How to Set One

The purpose of a boundary is twofold from my perspective:

1) Communicating what behavior you are willing to accept, and what behavior you are not willing to accept. This will cause you and the person you are setting boundaries with to be uncomfortable. Being uncomfortable is unavoidable when setting boundaries. See the uncomfortableness as a sign of success.

2) The other purpose for a boundary is to provide safety for you and whomever else you need to take care of.

When you set a boundary with an abuser, they're never going to say, "Gee, okay." They may *act* that way, but it's superficial. The abuser is going to manipulate the situation and try to avoid the pain or discomfort of the boundary. That's why you get nervous about setting one.

It's *extremely important* that *before* you set a boundary, you make it *abundantly* clear what it is you need. When you're in an

[9] HOW TO SET BOUNDARIES YOU CAN KEEP

abusive environment, one of the things that's very hard to have is clarity. This is because the person you're with is constantly blame-shifting, rationalizing, minimizing, justifying, and spiritualizing, leaving you in a state of internal confusion about what's really happening. Clearly understand what is happening when setting a boundary.

Clearly understand what is happening when setting a boundary.

How do you gain clarity about a boundary? Well, the first thing you've got to do is clearly understand what is happening. As we've talked about in this book, you've got to document what is happening so you can see your situation with complete clarity. Write about it honestly, without editing. Once you become clear, then you are ready to set a boundary. I encourage you to start small and resist the temptation to start with a hardcore boundary. It's tempting to start off with a big one because all you want to do is put an end to the pain you're in. But you must resist. There can be dire consequences for starting with too big a boundary. Allow change to happen by percentages. When someone is manipulative, it will be hard for them to keep whatever boundary you set. So I don't ever encourage victims of emotional abuse to set a boundary that they know cannot be kept.

Examples of a small boundary could be:

- Not giving him the benefit of the doubt in a situation.
- Saying no to something you don't want to do.
- Refusing to do things that are his responsibility.
- Being more honest with others about his behaviors behind closed doors.
- Taking time away for yourself.

Examples of a big boundary could be:

- Living separately.
- Confronting him about his harmful behaviors.

Boundaries must be effective in order to be healthy. For example, if you say, "I'm going to start detoxing from this relationship by never talking to him again." Well, that will almost certainly be an ineffective boundary because you won't be able to pull it off. Another example is telling your abuser, "I'm kicking you out!" And then for one reason or another you don't. In both cases, guess what you've communicated to your abuser? That *they* have the power, *not you*. You just gave them another mile by creating a boundary you cannot hold. As you document, write about what you believe is actually possible. Start by setting a small boundary that you can try, test, and use to gain strength.

I met with one client for five years. In the second session, I explained that her husband was not only abusive but was

[9] HOW TO SET BOUNDARIES YOU CAN KEEP

probably having multiple affairs based on the history she shared with me. "No, that's not possible," was her response. *Five years later*, after she had suffered a great deal of additional emotional torture, it came out that he'd not had just one affair, he'd had *nine*. Adding insult to injury, he had also been with prostitutes. You might think, *Finally, she has a smoking gun! She could set a boundary!* Unfortunately, that wasn't the case.

She had been so conditioned, trained, beaten down emotionally, and weakened internally that she had a very hard time setting any kind of boundary even *with* all of the evidence. I know from speaking with many people that setting a boundary is not an easy thing to do. Hold that in your mind. Setting a boundary is going to take time and support. You're going to need other people in your arena who can support you with whatever boundary you decide to set.

Everything in you is going to say no. You're going to try and find a way to rationalize away your reasons for setting the boundary in the first place. This is another reason to start small. Set a boundary you can hold. If you fail with your first boundary, that's okay. The effort was a good starting place. You can regroup and try again, but it's going to be hard.

When you start setting boundaries, you're going to cause pain. Your abuser has trained you throughout your entire relationship to not cause pain. If you've been attending church, then you've been trained that your job is to make people happy. You're supposed to love and care for them, not cause conflict or pain and be disruptive. You have been living with many internal, unconscious realities telling you to *not* set any boundaries.

---

*When you start setting boundaries,
you're going to cause pain.*

If any of the above examples represent what you're feeling or what you feel anxious about, then you're on the right track.

Case in point: One of the first ways I strongly encourage women in abusive relationships to set a boundary is in the bedroom. When you're in an emotionally abusive relationship, you are rarely interested in being intimate with the person who is harming you. Women have a strong internal desire to set a boundary that says, "No sex until you deal with *x, y, z*." Look for boundaries that you have some motive for and start there.

Remember, an abuser is going to try and manipulate to avoid the pain. Sometimes abusers will even react dangerously. You have to consider their possible reaction as you think about what you can handle.

I've confronted thousands of people in denial over the years while working in treatment and counseling. I've never told anyone who was in active denial the truth and had their first response be, "Oh gee, thank you. I appreciate the information." Abusers live in denial, as well as those whom they abuse. I have seen abusers respond to a boundary by agreeing to certain terms, but in their minds, they disagree and are furious about it but won't tell you. They respond with what

[9] HOW TO SET BOUNDARIES YOU CAN KEEP

they think you want to hear to avoid conflict and to avoid their own pain. They later act like you never said anything and thus continue the behavior. This is confusing and a blatant disregard of your needs.

Every person goes through this process differently. Every woman has their own strengths. Avoid the comparison game. When you're in the comparison game, you never win. Comparing yourself with others will always leave you feeling devalued. You'll never feel like you're on the winning side of the comparison game.

Take your situation as it is. Go back to the laser-like clarity you gained from painstaking documentation. Remember that one of the main things your abuser will do is try to prevent you from gaining clarity. But as you get clear, it leads to your freedom.

Setting boundaries is not an easy process. It's difficult, messy, and you're going to feel like you're turning yourself inside out. If you're having any of these feelings, *you're on the right track*. If it feels comfortable, you're probably being compliant and not causing your abuser enough discomfort.

Assess Your Safety Level

Before you go down the road of setting boundaries, you need to assess your safety level. Your abusive relationship may be with someone who is dangerous not only emotionally, but physically and financially too. They have the ability to take you out in one way or another. Your safety has to be a consideration, and I would *not* suggest you set a boundary with someone who is dangerous. Please, build a safety plan first *before* you move into the process of setting boundaries. Don't just fly off the handle and say, "I'm going to set a boundary!"

But how do you establish a safety plan? First, identify what your assets are. Who can help you? Do you have family members who understand and who have agreed to support you financially, emotionally? Can they also help with practical matters, such as housing or physical protection?

Assets can be relational and financial. It's important to know what yours are. Write them down. Documenting your assets will help you have clarity of mind as you step into the process of setting boundaries. That way, if things go sideways, you'll know what assets to pull from. Clarity can become very muddy once you've stepped into this process. You become disturbed and snap back into your pathology and training. You become reactive because that is what you've been trained to do for years.

Identify people who can speak into your world when you're spinning. Identify people you trust and listen to because they *are your assets.* Confronting your abuser by putting a boundary in place is an unavoidable part of the process. This confrontation is going to destabilize you, which is when you'll need to turn to your assets. Setting a boundary with your abuser is going to be one of the first major steps you'll take to becoming free. Setting a boundary is the opposite of avoidance. Boundaries you set are the process that leads you out and into

[9] HOW TO SET BOUNDARIES YOU CAN KEEP

your new life. As you set boundaries, one of two things is going to happen:

A. The abuser is going to prove his abusive ways by continuing the behavior.

B. They will (attempt to) change.

The probability of them changing is low. The probability of them manipulating with false change is very high. Firm boundaries will help you sift out what is real from what is false in their behavior. Remember, you're from Missouri now, the *show me* state. What they *do* is the most important thing, not what they say.

When you set a boundary, the abuser is immediately going to start using their words to try and manipulate you. He will come at you from different angles. Here's one angle I see abusers frequently attempt to use: For Candace and Dave, a boundary has been set that's severe and effective. In response, the abuser usually has some sort of epiphany. When Candace told her abusive husband, Dave, that he could no longer sleep in their bedroom or be intimate with her, he suddenly started reading his Bible more and became more involved at church. Being a good Christian was always part of Dave's public persona, but he upped his game after Candace set a severe boundary. The problem was his heart never changed. Dave's changes were cosmetic, not authentic.

If your husband has an "epiphany" like Dave's, it is actually an attempt to manipulate you from another angle. The abuser has changed tactics. Some might start using more biblical language or psychological terms. It's common for abusers to talk about their "epiphany" and how they're going to change. They claim they'll be the man you want them to be, love you the way *you need them* to love you … blah, blah, blah. Those are great words, and I hope those words prove to be true. Unfortunately, most often they're not. This is why you must pay close attention and evaluate the abuser's behavior. You must look past the false promises of change for *evidence* of real change through the abuser's behavior. You must continue to document the behavior that is harmful in the relationship in order to maintain clarity and make sure you hold that boundary.

Sometimes a boundary can mean a trial separation. This is one of my favorite things to help women do because once you get the abuser out, you can start to detox, as we discussed earlier. Detox is imperative for you to gain more clarity about your situation. By setting this particular boundary, you're able to evaluate their changes while providing safety and clarity for yourself.

As you start making more defined and immovable boundaries, you're going to experience difficulty. For example, Lisa and her husband, Tim, had a big argument last night. In the kitchen the next day, Lisa said, "You called me an offensive name in our argument yesterday. It was very hurtful."

Tim responded quickly, "No, I didn't. I don't know what *you heard*, but I didn't say that."

[9] HOW TO SET BOUNDARIES YOU CAN KEEP

After this defensive stance, Lisa set a clear boundary. "Look, I know what you said to me. I'm not going to allow you to gaslight me and tell me that what I heard wasn't real. This is one of many reasons why I don't trust you."

This is a clear boundary: *I'm not going to allow you to gaslight me and tell me what I heard wasn't real.* Lisa should expect to experience difficulty for setting this boundary. Your story will look different based on your unique situation.

To reiterate: Assess your assets to evaluate what you can do and what the limitations are. In your specific situation, you have to examine your assets very closely, then create a plan that is specific to your experience. Each person's situation is extremely nuanced and difficult, so there is no "one size fits all" approach.

Clearly defining *your* parameters for *your* specific situation will start to move you in a direction that's healthy for *you* but within *your* context. All of this is done with the goal of leading you to freedom, and that freedom is going to come in one of two ways:

A. The transformation of the abuser is effective and authentic.
B. The boundary you set gets them out of your life.

If your relationship is difficult because of an abuser, you have one of two goals. You either want to hurry up and destroy your relationship so that no one is harmed anymore, or you want to hurry up and heal it, so you can enjoy your lives.

However, that only happens when you clearly understand what you are and are not willing to accept. When you are being harmed on a regular basis, the most loving thing you can do is stop that person from harming you. *That really is the most loving thing you can do.* However, what you're told—especially women in our culture and specifically in the Christian culture—is that you're bad if you don't make the relationship work. You're not a loving wife. You're not a "good Christian." You're hardhearted, unforgiving, unkind … but the most loving thing you can do when someone is harming you is to *stop them*.

The most loving thing you can do when someone is harming you is to stop them.

Setting boundaries is loving. It's not hard-hearted. It's not mean-spirited. It's not cruel. It's loving. If that person transforms because you set a boundary, they will thank you. If they stay hard-hearted and continue being abusive, then you will spare your life and be able to live in a place of emotional health and safety. Your boundary will separate you from someone who is trying to destroy you internally.

SECTION III:
LIVE FREE

DEATH OF A THOUSAND CUTS

[10]

INTRINSIC VALUE

You Are Valuable.

HAVE YOU HEARD the term *intrinsic value*? This is the value you have simply because you exist. Let's think about this more deeply. Start by answering this question: From where do you get your value as a person? Many people in our culture get it from an outside source. They ask themselves questions, such as, "Do I have enough money? Do I have the right job? Do people look at me the way I want to be seen?" These are all external sources for value, which can easily be taken away.

But you are enough right where you are, right now, just because you exist. You are already valuable. What you do and how you behave doesn't affect your intrinsic value. Your actions affect your life experience, not your value.

Here's another way to understand intrinsic value. If you're driving down the road and see a car accident in which somebody got injured, do you stop and check to see if they are a criminal first before you help them? Do you weigh in your mind whether or not they're worth it? Or do you immediately, without thinking, dial 911 and try to help? Why is that our reaction to a human in need? Because life, in its very nature, is intrinsically valuable. You are valuable simply because you exist.

Life, in its very nature, is intrinsically valuable. You have intrinsic value simply because you exist.

Now, we need to give your circumstance some context. I've mentioned several times, in several chapters, how important it is to document what you are telling yourself in your mind, such as who you are and why you feel you're not good enough. Documentation was necessary so you could clearly see those negative, unproductive thoughts.

Now that you're headed in a positive direction, you have to do the same thing about your own value. Have you had any experiences in your life where your value was validated? Maybe someone treated you with kindness and respect? Has there been an event outside your ability to create but very

[10] INTRINSIC VALUE

much in your favor, maybe as if God was moving and showing Himself to you in a way you didn't ask for? It's very important that you document those things.

The committee in your mind that wags their collective finger at you is not going to be "pushed back" by something you don't know *for sure* is real. You must know in your soul that the truth is *really* true and *not* the lie. Otherwise, the committee is going to run you over, and you won't be able to live in the truth of your newfound freedom. Just because somebody lied to you, harmed you, and beat you down emotionally *doesn't mean you're less valuable*. It means you were harmed, it means you were hurt. I've been harmed and hurt, but that doesn't make me less valuable than the next person.

In our culture, and particularly in the Christian culture, we have all of these unspoken rules. If you don't look a certain way, act a certain way, have a certain level of strength or a certain level of *whatever*, then you're not okay. You're not valuable. You may have heard a "gospel" message that says, "God loves you *if* ..." This message says the value God gives you is based on whether or not you have done or believed all the right things. Ask yourself: *Do I really believe God values me based on whether or not I do or believe the right things? Whether or not I tithe, serve, witness, read the Bible, attend church regularly, or pray?* That is pure ammunition for the committee and only sets up an emotionally unhealthy value structure.

The Creator doesn't ever *devalue* life. He is the Author of life. The fact that you *have* life is a sign that He *cares* for you. He is motivated to be present with you, to reveal your value and help you see it. If there are people around you who can't or *won't* see your value, you have to put up boundaries. You will learn how to stop them from harming you because you are worth it. Your value is *profound*.

Documenting the positive, value-affirming circumstances that you've experienced is how you gain clarity. Those experiences that have caused you to feel and see your value become real when you write them down.

You could have had ten positive, value-affirming events in the last six months, but what will you remember? You will certainly remember the harm you've suffered during the same six months because the pain is right on the surface. Much of the positive-value events are just below the surface, so spend some time being quiet and letting yourself go back to those moments. Document when you felt them and how they made you feel by reliving them. When the committee in your head gets going, you're going to need something to look at and read.

That "wagging finger" confuses your thoughts, and you won't be able to slow it down or stop it. You need something that's written down so you can look at it and say, "Oh, that's right. On this date, this good thing happened. And on this date, that other good thing happened. Oh yeah! I remember this event." The events become almost tangible when they're written down. They're real events that you've experienced. The more you do this the more your sense of personal value will change to the positive. Eventually, you won't need to keep reading these events because they'll become part of you.

[10] INTRINSIC VALUE

That's how you fight back against the committee of voices in your head. By fighting back, you will be able to live in the freedom God gave you—the freedom that already exists.

Your value isn't something you have to go find. You already possess it. Allow yourself to see it, document it, and then live from it. After that, it's all about growing by percentages again. Let's say you live out of your value 1 percent of the time. If you move that to 1.1 percent of the time, your life will change radically. This is not about always being a happy-clappy person. This is about living in reality, and the reality is that *you are profoundly valuable.*

Sometimes, beginning to live out of your intrinsic value feels like a tectonic plate shift. Your whole world starts to change in both big and small ways when you move away from living in a devalued state and begin to realize your value. It can feel like you're being turned inside out. You're not quite sure what to do because the old system you're moving away from is what you're used to, it's what you know. The new system is something you don't know, so you're not so sure about what the future might hold. Living free means living in more uncertainty.

Living free means living in more uncertainty.

In order to live free, you have to live in more uncertainty. When you suddenly don't have someone abusing you, it often can feel destabilizing. Keep this in mind as you move through the process of living free and living out more out of your intrinsic value.

THE CHOICES ARE YOURS

You must start living out of your choice. You have a choice, and you must exercise it for your well-being, not because someone else has charge over you or because they get to tell you what to do. This can be a hard truth for people at church to grasp. The fact that God would say that women are not as valuable as men is *absurd*. Nevertheless, it has been falsely embedded in our culture, so it's another lie you will have to fight through.

I want you to hear that God is not upset with you for exercising your choices. In fact, it's His *profound mercy* that got you *out* of the abusive relationship.

[11]

NEW STANDARDS

YOU'VE SPENT YEARS in a very bad relationship where you've been abused. You've been undermined, you've been blamed as being the problem, and now you are pretty much emotionally destroyed. It's possible this scenario also played out in your childhood. In my childhood, I didn't have choices—I take that back—I had one choice: Comply or die. That was the rule system in my family. Whether your experience was like mine or not, something I see all the time among emotionally abused women is that when they go from not having *any* choices to suddenly living free, they feel wrong for even having a choice.

For example, there was a woman I'll call Mary who would change her clothes three, four, or five times a day because her husband, Steven, would see her and say, "Is that what you're wearing? What about the blue blouse? That shirt makes you look like a prostitute. What about the black jeans instead? Those jeans make you look fat."

And Mary would change her clothes again and again. Once she was free of Steven, she found it very unnatural and had some anxiety in choosing to wear whatever she wanted. Mary now had choices. No more of Steven's craziness. Mary later spoke to me about how wrong it felt for her to even be able to exercise her choice of the clothes she wore.

That seems odd, doesn't it? Feeling crazy for having a choice? But it's important to understand that on some level, this is going to happen to you. If you're making a choice and you feel slightly uncomfortable, you're in the right place. It's when you feel comfortable *not* making choices that you're in the abuse pattern again. You will ping-pong back and forth between making and not making choices. But don't worry. You're not going to stay that way.

You're going to go back and forth as you pursue living in freedom. That's how it works. Everything doesn't change all at once. God's mercy is that we change over time. There's no instantaneous change, which is why I never believe that when an abuser is confronted and has an epiphany that they're miraculously different the next day! You're being lied to because no one changes that quickly. Not even you.

God's mercy is that we change over time.

---

[11] NEW STANDARDS

RELATIONSHIPS POST-ABUSE

Let's take a look at your relationships *post abuse*. What if we replaced the foundational element of commitment with something else? In our culture and in the church, we are taught that the foundational element of marriage is commitment. What if we replaced commitment with intimacy and connection as the foundational element for a marriage? If you were healthily intimate and connected to another human being in a real, effective, and meaningful way, would commitment be an issue?

As you continue to move forward in your relationships, consider setting the standard as ...

1. Intimacy
2. Safety
3. Connection

One of the ways you're going to stay out of repeating the mistakes that got you into an abusive relationship in the first place is by setting those *new* standards as the bar that must be reached. In order to wind up in an abusive relationship, you had to devalue yourself, give up your choices, then listen to the other person rationalize, minimize, and justify their behavior by blaming you. In your post-abusive relationship, you don't have that faulty thinking, so you can say, "If Jim isn't going to be honest, caring, or emotionally intimate, then he's out."

Exercising your choices and living free keeps you out of dangerous relationships.

One of the number-one ways you're going to do this is by paying attention to your gut. You ended up in an abusive relationship because at some point you denied your gut. I've heard many people say that we deny the things we see in the abusive relationship for many reasons:

- To give the abuser the benefit of the doubt.
- To be compliant with our religious community.
- To make our parents happy.
- To not upset the kids.
- And so on.

We hear our gut say, "Hey. That's *not* okay." Then the committee in our head gets involved and talks us out of it. However, as you go through the process of living free, and while you pursue new relationships *after* the abusive relationship has ended, you will need to practice paying attention to your gut. As I've said before, if you act on your gut feelings just one out of ten times, you're going to have a big change in your life.

Trusting your gut will always cause your relationships moving forward to be healthier. You're going to have a higher level of internal, emotional, and spiritual freedom, which is

[11] NEW STANDARDS

what this whole process is about. You will be living free. When you live free, abusers can't be in your life.

*When you live free,
abusers can't be in your life.*

HEALTHY INTIMACY

You may be asking how it looks to live free in your intrinsic value within a new, healthy relationship? I've mentioned safe people, but how does that apply to the context of dating, or even the possibility of a more intimate, romantic relationship with someone? Well, because of a profound level of denial, the probability that an emotionally abusive man will successfully change is very low. Consequently, women who have gone through a divorce or the process of leaving an emotionally abusive man oftentimes need a new relationship. Add to this that hope in the *existence* of a good man may not be very high.

If you've been in an abusive relationship, you have seen yourself as the problem. You have seen yourself as not good enough because the message you received from your abuser was, "You're washed up, no good, and no one will *ever* want you. You're rotten goods, unredeemable." Those lies about your value are stuck in your head and give the abuser power. If you don't deal with the reality of those lies and start seeing someone new, you are setting yourself up for *another* abusive relationship.

As we've seen, living in freedom means you're living out of your intrinsic value. So when you're ready to begin a new relationship, it'll be very different because you know you have value. If a man you've started seeing does something unkind or undermining, your understanding of your intrinsic value says, "Next!" You're able to walk away and move on quickly before anything gets abusive. This is the opposite of what you practiced and how you lived in the abusive relationship, so it will feel like you're breaking some sort of cosmic rule. The problem is that when you don't have a strong understanding of your intrinsic value, you're very unsure.

One of the things that keeps people in an abusive relationship is a high priority on commitment. Women in the church culture have been told that it's *their job* to stay committed to the relationship. They're led to believe that if they don't stay, her husband will never change or heal. The burden is put on their shoulders to solve the abuse problem. You can't have that mindset, live free, and have a healthy relationship.

How do you move forward without commitment being the basis of your relationship? As I said before, moving intimacy and connection in to replace commitment as the basis of the relationship gives you a *choice*. Consequently, you start to live out of *your* choice.

You get to decide what to do with your life.

Remember the two rules:

[11] NEW STANDARDS

1) No crazy allowed.

2) You get to decide what is crazy.

Remembering these rules while dating is imperative. Learn to say, "No," and "I'm not interested." Now that you're no longer in an abusive relationship, you get to go through the process of discovering what it is *you* want. That's a beautiful thing. Unfortunately, the church culture often shakes its collective head and shames women for "checking it out." I often encourage women to date a lot because they have to discover who they are. Dating is part of the practice for *not* getting into an abusive relationship. Practice saying no when your gut tells you to, even when you can't explain it. Dating is practice for living free and trusting your gut without any guilt or strings attached. *It takes practice*, but much of the time there's a cloud around it like it's a bad thing. It's not.

I'm often asked if there are situations where women jump into dating too soon. Sometimes women turn to dating as a way to distract themselves from the pain of the loss of the relationship. My response to that is to cool down the grief a little bit *and* explore who you are. Instead of saying no, do both. The dating experience is going to move you forward and be a testing area for you to develop.

Another reality post-abusive relationship is that women are scared to ever trust another man. They often withhold themselves from relationships out of fear, which ends up further destroying their lives. I believe that no one is designed to live alone. People are designed to have connection. Yet it's still *your* choice how you move forward. You can choose to date or not to date, it's up to you.

One of the greatest tragedies of an emotionally abusive relationship is that you're in a relationship where you have all of the responsibilities and none of the benefits. You don't have any connection because the emotionally abusive person is in so much denial that they cannot connect. This is another reason why practicing dating could be beneficial for you.

Online dating is a way to practice being vulnerable in small ways without huge consequences. It can help you understand that you're actually okay. Being vulnerable is a good thing only in the presence of another human being who is safe enough to be vulnerable with. Be honest and trust your instincts.

Be honest and trust your instincts.

You might be thinking, *What if I end up getting manipulated again and don't see it coming? What if I end up dating another psycho?* It's no surprise if you're thinking these things and more. In fact, that's a *good* sign. It's healthy to realize you don't want a repeat of the past. I would hope not! The key for you to staying out of another abusive relationship is internal honesty and trusting your gut. Every woman I've ever talked to who got into an abusive relationship denied their gut in the beginning, then once it started happening, they denied it more and more. This is another reason why I think it is good to practice dating.

[11] NEW STANDARDS

When you have conflict in a relationship, you're either going to *gain* greater intimacy because of how the person handles it or *lose* intimacy because of how the person handles it. In an abusive relationship, the abuser is always telling you that *their* lack of ability to handle confrontation in a healthy manner is because of your inability to deal with it. It's *your* problem. When you're in a relationship with someone (friend, spouse, family member) who doesn't handle confrontation well, they can often become mean and divisive and start blame-shifting, denying, rationalizing, minimizing, justifying, and spiritualizing. This behavior separates us from intimacy. Again, in order to have intimacy, people have to exhibit *a lot* of healthy behavior.

Whether or not harm is going to happen in relationships isn't the main concern. You're dealing with human beings, so some form of harm is guaranteed. What's important is *how* the harm is handled. For example, if someone says something to you on a date that you don't like, pay attention to your gut and push back on what they've said. Respond by creating a boundary. Practice boundaries with that person who is not treating you well. That's how you can increase living in your intrinsic value. When you say no, what you're doing is valuing yourself. That's not what happened in the abusive relationship, but it is part of your new life of living free.

In the above, when I say "harm" we might also say "pain," but my purpose in using "harm" is to train you to recognize whether or not something someone says or does seems harmful and not just "playful" or factual" according to your gut. Most of us who have been subject to abuse have been taught and told that those moments "don't matter," or they were just "saying" or "kidding," to not take such things "too seriously," and that there is "no harm done" or intended and we are simply "too sensitive."

In chapter 5 we talked about trust and healing, and when somebody harms you and they then recognize and own it and make amends, that builds trust. But if someone's being harmful or unkind and they don't own it, then you need to set a boundary and move on, which is what I'm saying here, in particular with how this relates to creating and protecting healthy intimacy. We're now talking in the context of a relationship, about when, how, and why to set a boundary.

From now on, we will decide what's harmful and what's not. And what's important is how we handle the harm. We recognize it and set a boundary. We then see whether the other party owns it or not, which tells us what we need to know about them as a relationship partner. And in so doing, we set and protect a new higher standard for our relationship(s), and at the same time not only find but create our own intrinsic value.

[12]

RELATIONAL PARENTING

ONE OF THE most difficult situations that arises from being in an emotionally abusive relationship is parenting. There's nothing we value more than our kids. After you gain clarity about what's really happening in your life, you may see them being harmed too. What do you do? You want to make sure they can have a healthy life without being emotionally damaged. While it's a noble pursuit, it's not easy. It is very difficult for parents to be in a relationship with another person who is harming the children they both share.

In the process of parenting, ask yourself, "What do I want?" Do you want control, or do you want influence? With kids, control after about eight or nine years of age starts to vanish. You need to start letting go of control if your kids are getting beyond that age. Of course, this depends on the kid and how mature they are. However, our job as parents is *not* to control, it's to *influence*.

My way of controlling my kids was to homeschool them, but it came from my own history, trauma, and fear. *There is nothing wrong with homeschooling.* I want to make that perfectly clear. But I realize now that I was doing it out of fear. I was trying to prevent my kids from experiencing any harm. How on Earth could I ensure that my kids would *never* experience harm? It was a fool's errand.

When my kids were young, I used to stand over their beds and pray for them. I would say, "God, please don't let anything bad happen to them. Please, protect them."

God in my spirit would say, "So nothing bad happens to them, huh? You don't want them to grow?"

"Well, okay. Only allow the necessary harm that will help them grow."

God asked, "Have you looked around? Only the *necessary* harm is what happens to people?"

After that, my prayers changed. "God, please give me the grace to not lose my mind while they grow up."

The real issue was that I cared so much about them, I didn't want anything bad to happen. But bad stuff *is* going to happen. Being able to live in that reality instead of trying to prevent it is what makes parenting so difficult. This is what I mean by *relational parenting*. God Himself is a relational being. That's

[12] RELATIONAL PARENTING

what He wants us to be, and our job is to teach our kids how to be relationally healthy.

If you're in an abusive relationship, parenting is a very difficult task. You have one person exhibiting and teaching your children very *unhealthy* relational behavior, and you're left to try and manage the mess. To help get you through this, here are some tips to consider.

TELL THE TRUTH

I hear this all the time: "You should never bad-mouth the other parent." I agree with that, but in many cases, and particularly with emotional abuse cases, if you tell the truth about your spouse's behavior, will that make them look bad? Oh, yes. However, telling the truth isn't bad-mouthing. It's telling the truth.

What your kids don't know about what's going on will be made up in their heads. Kids make up things to fill in the blanks on their own until they hit puberty, which is when their hormones kick in. Puberty triggers brain development that allows the child to begin to distinguish between perception and reality. Prior to the development of that skill, they cannot separate the two.

Magical Thinking

Kids are capable of what's called "magical thinking." For example, two little boys are playing with G.I. Joe dolls, and you can hear them making gun noises: "Pew, pew, pew!" They mimic bombs exploding, trucks racing, helicopters flying, and so on. In their minds, everything is real because perception is king. It's their reality until they mature and can start to differentiate between what's real and what's perceived.

As the child is maturing, the abusive spouse gets into real trouble because the child starts to understand what's really going on. I'm sure you have heard this comment: "Everything was fine until my kids became teenagers, and then they lost their minds!" There's a scripture that says parents should "not exasperate your children."[10] It means do not be a hypocrite with your kids. Don't say one thing and then do another. Who respects a person like that? No one likes a hypocrite.

If you're behaving like that when your kids are in their early teens and learning how to distinguish between perception and reality, you're going to be in deep trouble. They're going to start to think, *Wait a minute. Mom and Dad said this, but they're doing that.* It breeds resentment, which only grows because you're being dishonest.

In relational parenting, you strive to stay connected with your children. This means you're going to have to live in some very uncomfortable realities. If you're in an emotionally abusive relationship, how do you handle watching your spouse

[12] RELATIONAL PARENTING

manipulate, shame, stonewall, gaslight, or harm your children? What are you supposed to do? Run in there and say, "You're abusing them! Get away!"

How do we work through all of that?

The number one thing to remember is you're going to be their mom for the rest of their lives. You have to play the long game. When you're in the abusive relationship, you often feel frantic and overwhelmed. You're constantly afraid because of the harm that's being done to your children, and you are worried about what they have to deal with. Then there's the pressure that *you* live in. So you're unhinged at times and have all this fear about the possible outcome. I understand all of that.

There is a way to navigate this emotional minefield.

BE PRESENT

Think about being connected and present with your kids as opposed to controlling or protective of them. If your spouse harms your kid and he or she says, "Mom, that really hurt," your best reply would be, "Yeah, I understand, honey. I know how hurtful that is. I'm with you." That's far better than saying, "Yeah, your dad's a jerk, and we should get away from him."

Right? Their dad *is* a jerk. And yes, you should get away from him. But what you need to do with the kid is *to be present*. You're modeling for them how to be a safe person and how to

DEATH OF A THOUSAND CUTS

be present. They will not see an example of this from the other parent.

There comes a time when you need to pull your kids out of an emotionally abusive environment. I've heard over and over that separation and divorce is "really hard on the kids, and they're going to be hurt." That's true, but if you keep your kids in an emotionally abusive home, they don't have *any* safe place to be.

Let's say you do separate or divorce your spouse because he won't change. And let's say your spouse gets unrestricted visits half the time, but the other half of the time the kids get a *healthy* parent—*you*. If you stay in the abusive relationship, they're not going to get that because you will be slowly destroyed and unable to be present with them. Being present with them is one of the most important things you can give your kids. I know that as a mom you're a nurturer, but you're going to have to fight that instinct to want everything to go well and to be good and safe. These are all good things, but let's be honest: You can't protect your kids from everything.

FACE REALITY

The best and most profound times I've had with my two kids have been up against the proverbial brick wall. I could see a brick wall coming a mile away because of my kids' behavior, immaturity, or lack of ability. When each wall was in view, I could have said, "Don't do that. You shouldn't do that." I could have tried to stop whatever was driving them toward the

[12] RELATIONAL PARENTING

brick wall. But I instead said, "Hey, I'm concerned about this," then they'd hit the brick wall. But later, they'd come to me and say, "So is this what you were talking about, Dad?"

"Mm-hmm," I said, nodding my head.

At that point they had internalized the lesson for themselves without me having to say anything.

> *The difference was in validating the truth instead of trying to install the truth.*

And it was all because I was present. That's called building relational credibility with your kids.

How are you going to spend your relational credibility? I would highly suggest that you *don't* spend your relational credibility trying to control or convince.

DROP IT AND ROLL

I want you to "drop it and roll" with your kids. You ask *one* question, get a response, and then move on to something completely innocuous. Or you make *one* statement of truth and then move on. For example: "Hey, honey, I know your dad said that. But it's not true. Now what would you like to drink?" Drop it and roll.

DEATH OF A THOUSAND CUTS

Wait and watch for moments to speak in this manner. Don't just try to dive into a subject and pull it apart. Drop it and roll. Your children will give you the opportunity at some point, but you need to be waiting for it. Then, when the opportunity comes, you can have a longer conversation.

No Unsolicited Advice

One rule I have for parents, particularly when dealing with kids in their teens and *especially* with adult children, is no unsolicited advice!

Zero, none, nada, zip.

You might be panicking right about now. I understand. I've got gold medals for unsolicited parental advice. I mean, come on! I know exactly what my kids should do, right? Here's why unsolicited advice is problematic: When you tell your child what they should do or give them advice without them asking, do you know what they hear?

"I'm not good enough."

"Mom doesn't like me."

"Mom thinks I'm inadequate."

I know that's not your intention, but that's what they hear.

You can make suggestions, but when your child asks you for advice, *that's when you give it and not before.* If your kids are under

[12] RELATIONAL PARENTING

ten, then as a mom, of course you have to tell them what to do and make sure they get their chores done. That's practical. But on an emotional level, you want to inspire relating safely with each other. You want to avoid controlling or fear-based interactions. Your job as a mom is to be relational in the moment, not raise outstanding citizens who have great relationships someday.

When you focus on *someday*, you are future-casting their lives instead of being present. When you future-cast their lives, whether you're conscious of it or not, you're developing an agenda and then relating to your children based on *your* agenda. When your child becomes your agenda, you stop loving them unconditionally because the relationship is now about you. If your behavior toward your child is driven by fear, your child will subconsciously realize that the relationship is about you and not them. That's where relational separation begins. Who wants to be around the person who is mainly concerned about themself?

However, if you've been documenting the emotional abuse and your resulting emotions, you'll be able to assess where you are emotionally, and you will know if you're able to listen and be present with your child. I know this is difficult because you're spending every minute defending yourself against your abuser. But as you become relational with your children, you are modeling a healthy way for them to live.

Kids do *not* do what you *say*, they *do* what you *do*. They pick stuff up by osmosis. Because they live with an abuser, they're inevitably going to pick up the abuser's tactics. There's no way around it, which is another reason why you have to clearly understand your situation, get to a safe place, and give them some context of how to be healthy.

I've said this before: Women sometimes can't leave their abuser for themselves but they *can* leave them for their kids. Whatever the reason, find the motive to help you get away from the abusive relationship or set the boundaries to protect yourself and others.

Do your best to stay relational, to stay noncontrolling, and to be present as much as possible. This requires you to get some space in your own world so that you're able to be present instead of sacrificing yourself in service of your kids. That is a noble distraction from the reality of the abuse, but it's still only a distraction. You may be telling yourself you're taking care of your kids, but what you're really doing is killing yourself, which is not good for them or for you.

Don't believe the lie that you don't matter. Do the internal emotional work so you can be relationally present with your kids, then present a living example of how to do that.

Be a relational parent and not a victim of abuse.

[12] RELATIONAL PARENTING

In Conclusion

In conclusion, breaking free from harmful relationships or situations can be very difficult, especially when you've been conditioned to believe the lies that you're not enough or that you don't have choices. But you do. You have the right to live a life that aligns with your true worth, and though it may feel daunting, trusting your gut is crucial in this process. When your gut tells you something is wrong, it's a signpost pointing you toward freedom and healing.

Understanding and embracing your intrinsic value is essential to living a life of freedom and wholeness. No harm, abuse, or mistreatment can diminish the profound value you inherently possess. The Creator has given you this worth, and it's time to recognize, embrace, and live from it.

As you grow in understanding your worth, your choices become clearer. You are worth a life filled with peace, joy, safety, respect, honesty, emotional support, affection, trust, and true love. This life aligns with the value you have always had and still today possess.

Remember, you are not less valuable because of what you've endured. You are resilient and have the power to make choices that lead to a life more aligned with your intrinsic value. Trust yourself—you are beautiful and worth it!

DEATH OF A THOUSAND CUTS

EPILOGUE:

THE POWER OF PRESENCE

I LIKE TO refer to the power of presence as the Holy Now. I can't take credit for this phrase. It was coined by the late pastor and author Eugene Peterson, whom I have an immense amount of respect for and who was a mentor to me through his writings. In a conversation I had with him, he said, "You cannot experience God or another human being at any other time but now, and now is a Holy place." It was a profound experience for me as I grabbed hold of this concept and began to learn what it truly meant.

Eugene Peterson has meant so much to me that I always tear up when talking about him. One of the things I've always appreciated about Eugene's books is he never tells you what to do. He simply writes about different topics and hopes the messages change you. The influence he's had on my life through his numerous writings has been transformational. So, sit with me for a moment. I want to share a story about Eugene. I had (and still have) a good friend named Jared, and we shared (and still share) a love of Eugene's writings. Like me, Jared began a personal transformation. We used to sit and talk for hours in Jared's sauna about Eugene's teachings and what we were learning. Sometimes one of us would bring our phone into the sauna so we could listen to passages of an audio book by Eugene. We would cry as we talked about the principles being revealed to us through his words.

As a guy who was abused and never cared for as a kid, the concept of *presence* eluded me. The level of friendship that Jared and I reached was only possible because of our shared experience with Eugene's writings. We came to a place of *real presence* with each other—the Holy Now—a place of high vulnerability and trust. One day, Jared had the crazy idea that we should meet Eugene.

"Yeah! Let's do that!" I said.

There are well-known videos online of Bono from U2 and Eugene discussing faith and the Psalms. These videos were filmed at the Peterson's home on Flathead Lake, Montana. Many times, I imagined myself sitting on their deck having numerous conversations about his books.[11] We wanted to fly to Flathead Lake and go door-to-door until we found him, but we decided we'd probably get arrested if we tried that.

So, what else could we do?

EPILOGUE: THE POWER OF PRESENCE

It was well-known Eugene Peterson loved receiving handwritten letters. He would always stop what he was doing and read each one as they arrived. In fact, one of his books is about him exchanging letters with people. So, we decided Jared would write Eugene a letter and we would fly to Montana. We were determined to meet Eugene. We overnighted Jared's letter and kept saying, "We're going to have a great time, and *maybe* Eugene will call."

After a few days in Montana with no call from Eugene, we decided we should probably just go sightseeing, that a visit with our favorite author probably wasn't going to happen. But not long after that, Jared received a call from Jan Peterson, Eugene's wife. If there had been a camera in that room, the world would have seen two grown men dancing around, yelling and screaming, "We're going to meet Eugene!"

We arrived at Eugene's property and while walking down the hill could see his house and deck, where Eugene was sitting, reading a book. It was unbelievable! It almost took my breath away. I had that exact picture in my mind so many times. He spoke to us about his love of Montana, its beauty, and how good it was for his soul. With his wife, the four of us talked for over three hours. In one amazing moment, Jared read Eugene the letter he had written, asking if we could meet him. In it, Jared said we would be glad to take him and his wife to dinner or to meet them anywhere they liked. Jared wrote that Eugene had powerfully changed him. He explained he had been harmed by his father, and that Eugene had been a father to him through his writings. Eugene became very emotional. It was spiritually meaningful and powerful.

DEATH OF A THOUSAND CUTS

To see him cry when we told him how much he meant to us because of his writings is something I'll never forget. A few months after that conversation, Eugene died. To this day, I know I was given the incredible privilege of time with that influential man. All the emotion that came out as a result of the meeting with Eugene shows the power of presence. Gratefully, I have experienced the Holy Now of presence both in my relationship with Jared and with Eugene, personally and through his books.

I'm very fortunate to have had it all come full circle at his home, on his deck, overlooking Flathead Lake in a tearful conversation of gratitude.

It was a long process for me to learn how to trust and be vulnerable with another human being. So, to reach the level of vulnerability I had with Jared and to then be able to sit with Eugene on his deck was beautiful. What I learned about presence and relationship prompted me to start a church based on Eugene's writings of the subject. A pastor's job is to be *with* the people. It's not necessarily to teach and preach. Teaching and preaching are important, but real change happens when you are relational and *present* with a person. The church I pastored was based on this concept, and it was life-changing.

ABOUT THE AUTHOR

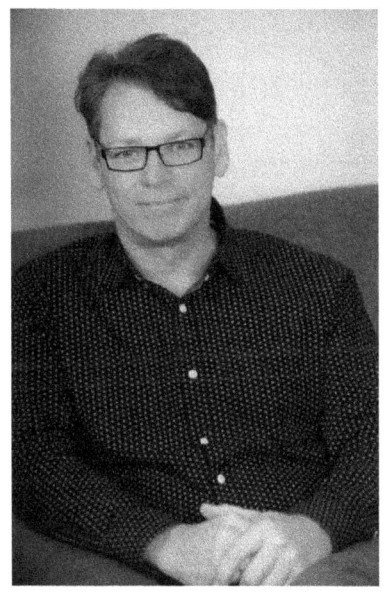

PATRICK DOYLE, a seasoned counselor with over three decades of experience, has devoted his career to guiding individuals toward a life free from the chains of harm, empowering them to recognize their intrinsic value. He has become a trusted voice and leading expert in the realm of emotional and spiritual trauma. Patrick is the founder and visionary behind Pathway to Hope, an online program dedicated to supporting women to navigate the complexities of emotional and spiritual abuse.

Beyond his impactful work, Patrick cherishes his role as a father to his two grown sons. He also indulges his love for the Braves as an avid baseball fan.

To delve deeper into Patrick's insights and resources, visit his website at www.PatrickDoyle.life.

DEATH OF A THOUSAND CUTS

IF YOU OR SOMEONE YOU KNOW IS IN AN ABUSIVE SITUATION, PLEASE REACH OUT FOR HELP. THE NATIONAL DOMESTIC VIOLENCE HOTLINE IS AVAILABLE 24/7 AT:

1-800-799-SAFE (7233)

OR BY TEXTING START TO 88788.

WEBSITE: HTTPS://WWW.THEHOTLINE.ORG/

DEATH OF A THOUSAND CUTS

GLOSSARY

Terms as Used by Patrick Doyle
& Pathway to Hope

arranged alphabetically

---

blame-shifting
    The manipulative tactic used by an abuser to deflect responsibility for their harmful actions or behavior onto the victim. Blame-shifting involves attributing fault, guilt, or responsibility to the victim for the problems in the relationship or for the abusive behavior perpetrated by the abuser. This can include making the victim feel responsible for the abuser's anger, justifying abusive actions by citing the victim's behavior, or minimizing the abuser's actions while magnifying the victim's perceived faults. Blame-shifting in an emotionally abusive relationship undermines the victim's sense of self-worth, perpetuates feelings of guilt and shame, and maintains the abuser's power and control.

codependence
    "External dependence," the process of your soul and your value as a person becoming dependent on external realities. External dependance is defined as someone who derives their value as a human being based on whether other people approve of them or not. Value comes from outside sources instead of being generated from within oneself.

connection
    The deep bond and resonance that individuals share with each other, characterized by a profound understanding, empathy, and shared emotional experiences. Emotional connection goes beyond surface-level interactions and involves a genuine attunement to each other's feelings, needs, and perspectives. It is built on mutual trust, respect, and vulnerability, allowing individuals to feel seen, heard, and valued by their partner. Emotional connection fosters a sense of intimacy,

belonging, and support in relationships, enhancing communication, empathy, and overall relationship satisfaction.

denying

The deliberate refusal or dismissal of the experiences, feelings, or needs of the victim by the abuser. Denying involves invalidating the victim's reality, gaslighting them into questioning their perceptions, memories, or sanity. This can manifest as denying the occurrence of abusive incidents, minimizing their impact, or shifting blame onto the victim. Denying in an emotionally abusive relationship serves to maintain control over the victim, perpetuate the cycle of abuse, and undermine their sense of self-worth and agency.

disregarding (ignoring)

The intentional act of dismissing the needs, emotions, boundaries, and well-being of the victim by the abuser. Disregarding/ignoring involves refusing to acknowledge the victim's presence, feelings, or concerns, and actively avoiding engagement or validation. This can manifest as ignoring the victim's attempts to communicate, withholding affection or attention, or invalidating the victim's experiences and perceptions. Disregarding/ignoring in an emotionally abusive relationship serves to undermine the victim's sense of worth, isolate them emotionally, and maintain control over the relationship dynamics.

gaslighting

The psychological manipulation tactic used by an individual, often in an abusive relationship, to undermine another person's perception of reality, memory, or sanity. Gaslighting involves denying the victim's experiences, feelings, or observations, and intentionally causing them to doubt their own thoughts, judgments, or sanity. This can include distorting the truth, fabricating information, or trivializing the victim's concerns, making them feel confused, insecure, or dependent on the gaslighter for validation or approval. Gaslighting is a form of emotional abuse that aims to maintain power and control over the victim by eroding their self-confidence, autonomy, and sense of reality.

GLOSSARY

ignoring
    (see disregarding)

intimacy
    The deep connection and bond between individuals characterized by a mutual sense of trust, vulnerability, and understanding. Emotional intimacy involves the ability to share one's innermost thoughts, feelings, and experiences with another person in a safe and supportive environment. It encompasses open communication, empathy, and acceptance, allowing individuals to feel fully seen, heard, and valued by their partner. Emotional intimacy fosters a sense of closeness, security, and emotional fulfillment in relationships, contributing to greater intimacy, connection, and resilience in the face of challenges.

justifying
    Providing excuses, explanations, or rationalizations for the abusive behavior of the perpetrator, often aimed at convincing the victim and others the behavior is acceptable or justified. This can involve blaming the victim for the abuse, minimizing the severity of the actions, or distorting reality to make the abuse seem warranted. Justifying in an emotionally abusive relationship perpetuates the cycle of abuse by undermining the victim's perceptions, manipulating their sense of reality, and reinforcing the power dynamics that allow the abuse to continue.

minimizing
    The manipulative tactic used by an abuser to downplay, dismiss, or invalidate the emotions, experiences, concerns, or autonomy of the victim. This can involve belittling the victim's feelings, needs, or perspectives, making them feel insignificant or unworthy. Minimizing may also entail trivializing or rationalizing the abuser's harmful behavior or actions, making excuses, or shifting blame onto the victim. Overall, minimizing serves to maintain control over the victim, undermine their self-esteem, and perpetuate the cycle of abuse.

raging
    The use of derogatory language, insults, or verbal attacks by one partner towards the other, aimed at demeaning, belittling, or humiliating them. This form of emotional abuse can include name-calling, mockery, ridicule, or criticism intended to undermine the victim's self-esteem and confidence. Ragging is often used as a means

of exerting power and control over the victim, creating an atmosphere of fear, intimidation, and emotional distress. It serves to diminish the victim's sense of worth and agency within the relationship, perpetuating a cycle of abuse.

rationalize

To attempt to explain or justify one's behavior, beliefs, or decisions in a way that makes them seem rational or logical, despite being harmful.

safety

The feeling of security, comfort, and trust that individuals experience in their relationships and environments, knowing that their emotional well-being will be respected, valued, and protected. Emotional safety is characterized by an absence of fear, judgment, criticism, or harm, allowing individuals to freely express their thoughts, feelings, and vulnerabilities without the fear of rejection, ridicule, or retaliation. It involves establishing healthy boundaries, fostering open communication, and cultivating empathy and understanding. Emotional safety promotes a sense of stability, connection, and intimacy in relationships, contributing to overall psychological well-being and resilience.

spiritualizing

The manipulation tactic employed by an abuser to exploit spiritual beliefs, practices, or values in order to control, manipulate, or justify their abusive behavior. This can involve distorting religious or spiritual teachings to assert dominance over the victim, using scripture or spiritual concepts to justify abusive actions, or coercing the victim to comply with the abuser's demands under the guise of spiritual authority. Spiritualizing in an emotionally abusive relationship often involves exploiting the victim's faith or spirituality to maintain power and control, while undermining their sense of autonomy and self-worth.

LEARN MORE

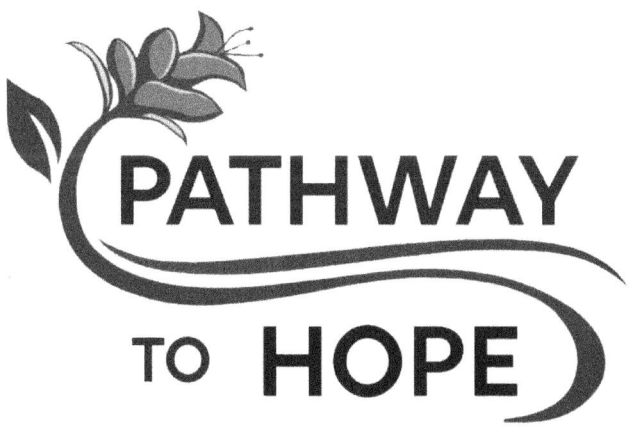

Learn more about the Pathway to Hope Course.

Visit www.PatrickDoyle.life

DEATH OF A THOUSAND CUTS

NOTES

[1] https://www.azquotes.com/author/11465-M_Scott_Peck/tag/pain

[2] Agape, in the New Testament, the fatherly love of God for humans, as well as the human reciprocal love for God. In Scripture, the transcendent agape love is the highest form of love and is contrasted with eros, or erotic love, and philia, or brotherly love. —https://www.britannica.com/topic/agape

[3] Emotional abuse can happen in any kind of relationship, not just romantic relationships. In this book I use "partner" to describe the person with whom you're in an emotionally abusive relationship.

[4] Many churches and pastors interpret Ephesians 5:22–33 in a way that enables men to have complete control over their wives and families. When this domineering understanding of marriage is taught, the idea of divorce becomes intolerable, even unspeakable in some cases. You'll be told to just forgive him and keep the marriage together and to not even think of separation or divorce. This makes marriage an idol. The marriage itself becomes more important than the safety and health of those within it. The Life-Saving Divorce is a well-researched book by Gretchen Baskerville. It is a helpful resource for understanding marriage and divorce differently.

[5] In this book, I use the word "intimacy" to mean a safe, mutual, healthy emotional connection.

[6] 1 John 4:16 ESV

[7] Proverbs 31: 10-31, New International Version
Epilogue: The Wife of Noble Character
10 [b]A wife of noble character who can find?
  She is worth far more than rubies.
11 Her husband has full confidence in her

DEATH OF A THOUSAND CUTS

    and lacks nothing of value.
12 She brings him good, not harm,
    all the days of her life.
13 She selects wool and flax
    and works with eager hands.
14 She is like the merchant ships,
    bringing her food from afar.
15 She gets up while it is still night;
    she provides food for her family
    and portions for her female servants.
16 She considers a field and buys it;
    out of her earnings she plants a vineyard.
17 She sets about her work vigorously;
    her arms are strong for her tasks.
18 She sees that her trading is profitable,
    and her lamp does not go out at night.
19 In her hand she holds the distaff
    and grasps the spindle with her fingers.
20 She opens her arms to the poor
    and extends her hands to the needy.
21 When it snows, she has no fear for her household;
    for all of them are clothed in scarlet.
22 She makes coverings for her bed;
    she is clothed in fine linen and purple.
23 Her husband is respected at the city gate,
    where he takes his seat among the elders of the land.
24 She makes linen garments and sells them,
    and supplies the merchants with sashes.
25 She is clothed with strength and dignity;
    she can laugh at the days to come.
26 She speaks with wisdom,
    and faithful instruction is on her tongue.
27 She watches over the affairs of her household
    and does not eat the bread of idleness.
28 Her children arise and call her blessed;
    her husband also, and he praises her:
29 "Many women do noble things,

[12] THE POWER OF PRESENCE

> but you surpass them all."
> 30 Charm is deceptive, and beauty is fleeting;
>   but a woman who fears the Lord is to be praised.
> 31 Honor her for all that her hands have done,
>   and let her works bring her praise at the city gate.

Footnotes: Proverbs 31:10 Verses 10-31 are an acrostic poem, the verses of which begin with the successive letters of the Hebrew alphabet. (https://www.biblegateway.com/passage/?search=Proverbs+31&version=NIV)

(Notes continued)

[8] mainline, intransitive verb. (1) To inject (an illegal or addictive drug, such as heroin) directly into a major vein. (2) To inject a drug intravenously. —From *The American Heritage® Dictionary of the English Language, 5th Edition.*

[9] Peck, M. Scott. *The Road Less Traveled, Timeless Edition: A New Psychology of Love, Traditional Values and Spiritual Growth.* Touchstone, 2003.

[10] Ephesians 6:4.

[11] Eugene Peterson and Bono, "The Psalms," https://www.youtube.com/watch?v=-l40S5e90KY.

www.ingramcontent.com/pod-product-compliance
Lightning Source LLC
Chambersburg PA
CBHW070625030426
42337CB00020B/3914